THE WELLNESS WAY TO WEIGHT LOSS

THE WELLNESS WAY TO WEIGHT LOSS

Elizabeth M. Gallup, M. D.

Springer Science+Business Media, LLC

Library of Congress Cataloging-in-Publication Data

Gallup, Elizabeth M.
The wellness way to weight loss / Elizabeth M. Gallup.
p. cm.
Includes bibliographical references and index.

1. Reducing diets--Recipes. 2. Nutrition. I. Title.
RM222.2.G343 1990
641.5'635--dc20 90-41746
CIP

ISBN 978-0-306-43568-3 ISBN 978-1-4899-6295-9 (eBook)
DOI 10.1007/978-1-4899-6295-9

The recipes for microwave cooking on pages 139–199 are taken with permission from *Microwaving Light & Healthy,* © 1985 Cy DeCosse Incorporated.

The recipes on pages 200–213 are reprinted by courtesy of The Quaker Oats Company.

Originally published by Plenum US in 1990.
Softcover reprint of the hardcover 1st edition 1990

Acknowledgments

Many individuals aided in the preparation of this book; I thank them all. Special appreciation goes to Cindy Elliott for her encouragement, Marty Litherland for her brilliance, Melissa Cilley for her endurance, Janan Juliff for her tolerance, Lisa Miller for her diligence, and special thanks to my patients in Defiance, Ohio. This book is dedicated to their Wellness.

Contents

1

America, the Land of Plenty

One out of every four Americans is 20 percent or more overweight. Thirty percent of all women wear a size 14 or larger dress. The average American goes on 24 weight loss diets during his or her lifetime. Recently, statistics revealed that there are 50 million people in America on a diet and another 50 million who want to go on one. All of these observations demonstrate that America—"the land of plenty"—is plenty fat.

Being overweight has a great negative impact on health, not to mention the negative effect it produces psychologically. Of the 37 percent of adults in the United States who are on diets, only 3 percent manage to lose weight and keep it off. Living in America, where food is easy to get and consume, has helped us gain excess weight. This revolutionary diet book not only will assist you in losing weight but will also be your guide to staying or becoming well at the same time. This is the Wellness Way to Weight Loss.

WHY IS THIS DIET BOOK UNIQUE?

This is one of the most unique diet books ever written. Why? Because not only is it a book that will enable you to lose weight; it is also a Wellness book. Wellness is the pursuit of happy, healthy living. It is a way of life—not just a diet. After applying the Wellness Way to Weight Loss diet to your everyday routine, it will become second nature. You will never have to diet again.

One aspect of Wellness is to be of optimal weight. Not only will this book teach you how to lose weight, but the guidelines you learn will enable you to keep weight off permanently.

Also unique to the concept of Wellness is that it provides guidelines applicable to everyone. How many of you remember all those countless diets you tried while your family complained that they were being starved? Or how many times have you been on a diet but couldn't even eat with your family because the diet was so restrictive? How many times have you been on a diet and felt ill or sickly? The Wellness diet is one that all of us can follow to lead happier and healthier lives. Eating the Wellness way will soon become natural to you if you follow its guidelines. You will look better and feel better.

In addition to the unique incorporation of Wellness concepts, this book also includes the latest developments in diet and exercise literature. These developments include a description of the amazing ability of carbohydrates and fiber foods to help you lose weight. The value of these components in our diet is only beginning to be understood.

Another important aspect of the Wellness Way to Weight Loss diet is its variety. Often, the diets that are heavily advertised (the fad diets for which you usually pay an enormous amount of money) are too restrictive. Sure, while you are on them you lose weight, but because they are so boring you can't stick to them. Or, after you have lost your weight, you go off them and, boom, all the weight is gained back and more. Or you feel so sickly you crave much more food. This happens because your body hasn't learned anything on the diet. You haven't changed your eating habits and you haven't learned how to eat well. As a result, such diets don't work or they do work but only temporarily. The Wellness Way to Weight Loss diet works and lasts because it is a new, enjoyable, and healthy way to eat. Not only are you eating food that is good for you; you are also losing weight. There is so much food to choose from that you cannot possibly become bored.

Even after you lose weight and are happily maintaining your desired weight, you will inevitably stray off the road of Wellness. We all do. But know that you will return to good eating habits because they will be familiar to you and you will know the benefits that can be reaped from doing so.

THIS BOOK IS WRITTEN BY A DOCTOR

I am a family physician with a very active practice. Day after day I counsel patients in my office regarding weight loss and Wellness. Week after week I give innumerable talks around the country regarding Wellness and weight loss. The Wellness Way to Weight Loss is what I advocate because it works. In my practice I repeatedly see patients who come to me for advice on how to lose weight. I teach them the same principles that you will find here.

Not only has the Wellness Way to Weight Loss worked for my patients but it has worked for me as well. In 1986 I decided to run a marathon and participate in triathlons—two grueling events requiring great physical endurance. I read the literature on diets for athletes and participated in a conference on Wellness. Some of the information was from well-known sources such as the American Heart Association and the American Dietetic Association. Other information was from medical and nutritional literature. I put all of the information together and found that the only thing in diet literature that works is something that is somewhat familiar to all of us. All of the information was there but had not yet been brought together in one place. This book represents the synthesis of that information.

I combined these familiar principles in a single, new, compact, and applicable program and completed a 26.3-mile marathon. In addition I competed in and won several triathlons. I knew that I had to lose weight to be competitive. I accomplished that weight loss by following my own guidelines, which are incorporated here. Since then, I have used the same model on a daily basis with my patients. My impetus to lose weight was my desire to be competitive. Certainly you won't be expected to run marathons or triathlons after reading this book, but the concepts and principles of losing weight, and looking and feeling better, are the same regardless of your motive.

The Wellness Way to Weight Loss is *the* definitive way to lose weight, and it is *the* definitive way to keep weight off. Never has any discussion of diet concepts been so applicable to everyday life. Never have so many familiar weight-loss principles been assembled together in one publication. The Wellness Way to Weight Loss provides you with complete information both about losing weight and with the basic principles of keeping a healthy diet. These concepts can be applied on a daily basis in your home because the same diet you are on is one your family can also enjoy.

WHAT THIS DIET TALKS ABOUT

This weight loss program is a multifaceted diet. It includes basic nutritional guidelines which are not only used to lose weight but can also be applied to your daily diet routine after you have reached your optimal weight. These nutritional principles will be carried with you for the rest of your life, so that weight gain will not be a problem again.

Each chapter specifically addresses a component of either good nutrition, exercise, or both. It is important for you to read each chapter. The information contained in the chapters will get you on the road to healthier eating and successful weight loss. Now, go forth, learn, enjoy, and *lose weight*—the Wellness Way.

2

Wellness

What Is It?

Wellness is the pursuit of happy, healthy living. Wellness reflects the fact that you alone as an individual are responsible for your own health. Wellness is a way of life that incorporates good health habits and is defined within the context of taking care of yourself. In Wellness, you are not only taking care of yourself in a physical sense but also in a nutritional, spiritual, and emotional sense. In other words you assume care for yourself in all areas of your life. If you work toward a "well" life-style, then you will develop habits that support a pattern of living guided by positive benefits. This new life-style will promote an overall sense of well-being.

A Wellness life-style is available to anyone who is willing to seek it. It is free of charge—anyone who wants it can afford it. Wellness depends only upon your motivation as an individual.

The Wellness movement has swept America. Patients are demanding more than just "sick care" from their physicians. They are demanding evaluation, motivation, and education in how to take care of themselves so they can lead vibrant, more fulfilling lives.

Unfortunately, few doctors know very much about Wellness. The model taught in medical schools is the treatment of disease. Very little time is devoted to disease prevention or nutrition and exercise. However, this is gradually changing as more and more patients are beginning to understand the importance of Wellness and more and more medical students are demanding a better education in the Wellness areas.

WHY THE INTEREST IN WELLNESS?

Why have we become so interested in Wellness lately? One of the chief causes is the skyrocketing cost of medical illness. By 1981, 10 percent of the nation's gross national product, over $297 billion, went toward the treatment of disease. As a nation we spend more on health care costs than we spend on either defense, education, or welfare. General Motors spends more today in health care costs for employee benefits than for steel to make its new cars.

Industry has made a big push toward Wellness. Sick employees cost industry a great deal of money, while Wellness programs decrease the number of sick employees and reduce absenteeism, thereby saving money. Furthermore, employees who are well have a greater commitment to the organization, and the efficiency of their work improves markedly over those who are not well. Recently, poor nutrition has become a real concern to industry. Losing an employee can be very costly. The industry has to retrain another person to perform the last employee's job. The person who is 20 percent overweight increases his or her chances of an early death by 20 percent. If a person is more than 20 percent overweight, the chance of premature death jumps to 50 percent. Preventing such a loss is a cost-effective policy for the spending of corporate dollars.

The interest in Wellness is apparent in a recent survey of Americans taken by *Psychology Today*. Results indicated that physical health has taken on great importance in the lives of Americans, many of whom spend more time thinking about health than love or money. Furthermore, the survey found that 57 percent of the respondents participate in fitness programs. Finally, the survey showed that a large percentage of Americans are concerned about nutrition, with 4 out of 10 people avoiding salt and a third of all people avoiding sugar.

A recent Gallup poll showed that 81 percent of all Americans believe that being in good health is very important and ranks second only to the importance of a good family life. With the quest for health comes corresponding benefits of a youthful appearance and the feeling that you are in charge of your own body, both of which serve as continuing motivational forces for Wellness.

THE EVOLUTION OF WELLNESS

The term Wellness emerged in the 1960s. However, the actual word has its roots in the early Greek and Oriental civilizations. The ancient philosophers and physicians set forth principles that were, and still are, basic to good health. These early thinkers observed the interaction between the human being and his or her environment, including the social, emotional, occupational, and spiritual environments. Even back then there was a correlation between the environment and health. Bad environment equals bad health and vice versa.

Hippocrates derived some early principles that are also found in the writings of early Chinese physicians. These writings include the following:

1. Health is a state of balance. Illness represents imbalance and is a natural phenomenon. It then can be studied and influenced by therapeutic procedures and wise management of a person's life.
2. The onset of illness can be correlated with abrupt changes in the environment.
3. Mind, body, and environment are interdependent.
4. Nature has inherent healing powers. The physician has a responsibility to create the most favorable conditions in which healing can occur.

So, from the time physicians and philosophers started observing human behavior and disease, a link was noted between what was happening around us and what was happening to our bodies. Up until the late 1800s, health was valued as a process that needed to be worked for in the same manner that any goal is actively pursued. Illness was perceived as an imbalance between the individual and the world.

However, in the late 1800s the germ theory of medicine was founded. The germ theory proposed that disease could be attributed not to the individual's imbalance but to an external force—germs—outside the body over which the ill person supposedly had no control.

This shift to the germ theory also brought about a shift in the approach to health. The new approach transferred the individual's responsibility for his or her own health to "something else." This way of thinking continued until the early 1960s and is still quite prevalent today. It is easier to blame conditions like obesity, illness, and general poor health on anything and everything when the real culprit is often as controllable as unhealthy life-style habits. Certainly not all diseases are caused by poor life-style habits, but it has been shown that such habits increase the risk of developing certain diseases. Poor life-style habits also have a tendency to worsen certain diseases such as high blood pressure and diabetes.

The Wellness movement which began to emerge in the 1960s and 1970s started to shift the focus back toward the individual's responsibility for his or her own health. Once again, life-style started being linked to disease. The Surgeon General finally said unequivocally that smoking causes cancer. Health care professionals began looking at the reasons people had died over the last 10 to 20 years, and causes of death began to be associated with the life-styles the persons had led.

Because of this new information relating life-style choices such as smoking, obesity, and the excessive use of alcohol to disease, people began to modify their life-style habits. They began to get *well*. Studies such as Harvard's Framingham Study about the connection between health and life-styles, along with information about the decline in heart attacks associated with jogging, prompted people to become interested in learning how to get and stay well.

As a result of the awakened interest in Wellness, studies were undertaken to examine the costs of bad life-style habits such as smoking, drinking, and overeating. Industries were very interested in these cost studies because they clearly demonstrated that bad life-style habits cost them money. Consequently, some companies began to offer their employees Wellness programs.

So, as we can see, there has been a major shift back to the original way of thinking—Wellness is a way of living that promotes and supports health. Certainly individuals, and their physicians, should be aware of the impact germs can have on their well-being, but the concept that each of us has the ability and the responsibility to make choices affecting our own health has laid the groundwork for the growth of the Wellness movement.

Wellness not only enables you to live longer; it can actually help you live better. You will feel better, be more committed to your job, and generally be more satisfied and content with your life. And best of all, your quality of life will increase dramatically. Wellness is life-enhancing and within your reach.

3

The Fat Stat

You probably know people who can eat constantly and never seem to gain weight. While in medical school, I rented a cottage at the beach with five of my classmates. For one long week I had to live with someone who had that envious ability to eat all the time and still remain thin. My classmate not only ate a bigger breakfast than all of us, she also ate two doughnuts between breakfast and lunch, enjoyed a huge lunch, snacked all afternoon, and ate dinner. She never, ever skipped dessert. I ran 3 miles a day; she was lucky if she walked two. I did everything I could not to hate her.

What I have since come to learn is that her body had decided how much it wanted to weigh; no matter what she ate, she remained at the weight her body had chosen for her. This decision by the body to weigh a certain amount has been called various things, two of which are the *setpoint* and the *fat thermostat*. I like to call it the "Fat Stat." Fat because obviously when you think of weight you think of fat, and stat because stat is derived from the word *static* which means stationary or in equilibrium. This is the way our body behaves. It decides, and we don't know why, to weigh a certain amount, and once the weight is set, the body tries to keep that amount the same, or static. So if your body has decided to weigh 10 pounds more than you want it to, losing those 10 pounds permanently will require that you change your Fat Stat. If you are lucky and your body has set its Fat Stat just where you want it to be, then you probably can eat just about anything you want (within reason, of course) and maintain the weight you want.

Let me illustrate this concept in another way. Take two women who are exactly the same age, the same height, and have the same bone structure—that is, both are medium framed. One woman may be able to eat 2500 calories a day and never gain weight, while the second woman may only be able to eat 1000 calories a day; any more and she gains weight. This is so because the Fat Stat on the woman who can eat anything she wants is set at a lower weight—a lower setpoint than the second woman. The woman who can eat a lot of calories has an inefficient engine. She supplies it with energy in the form of calories, and because her body's engine is so inefficient it doesn't store any of the calories; it uses all of them up. But the second woman has a very efficient engine which doesn't need many calories to run, and the extra calories are stored as fat.

To lose weight effectively you must lower your Fat Stat. To lower your setpoint requires lower calories and increased exercise. Exercise is a form of energy output that can be understood to arise from three different mechanisms. The first mechanism is *basal metabolism*, which is your baseline energy level or the rate you burn up calories at rest. The second factor in energy output is *thermogenesis*, which is energy that you give off in the form of heat, or energy above the basal metabolic rate. Finally, the third form of energy output is *exercise*. All energy causes you to expend calories.

The only other way to modify the Fat Stat will be to change your rate of thermogenesis. The factors contributing to thermogenesis are food intake and exposure to temperatures below body temperatures. Your body expends more calories digesting certain types of food than others. For example, your body spends more calories digesting carbohydrates than fat (discussed in greater detail later). Therefore, to increase your thermogenesis and your energy expenditures, it is better to eat more carbohydrates than fat. The more energy you expend, the more weight you lose. The second part of thermogenesis, exposure to cold temperatures, causes you to expend energy because your body is generating heat to keep warm. This is not to say that a good way to lose weight is to run naked in the snow, but heat production uses energy.

One of the most exciting developments in diet literature is the investigation of thermogenic drugs. These drugs increase the level of heat given off above the basal metabolic rate. By taking one of these drugs, your Fat Stat would be lowered. Unfortunately, these drugs are still being tested and are not yet available.

So, you see, the Fat Stat governs what you will weigh and also explains why some people eat and eat and stay thin, while others starve and are fat. In fact, most overweight people have a setpoint which causes them to be efficient users of calories so that they stay at a higher weight: they have a higher Fat Stat. An easy way to understand this concept is higher Fat Stat equals higher weight, lower Fat Stat equals lower weight. The goal of the Wellness Way to Weight Loss is to lower the Fat Stat.

The Fat Stat is one of the key elements in weight loss. The bad news for some unsuccessful dieters is that the Fat Stat is given to them like the color of their eyes. Your individual Fat Stat is very dependent on your parents' history. If your mother always had a weight problem, she probably had a high Fat Stat. The good news is that your Fat Stat can be changed to some degree. It must be reset in order for you to lose weight and, more important, to keep it off. The next chapter will discuss in detail how the Fat Stat is intertwined with successful dieting and how it sabotages many attempts at weight loss.

4

The Ups and Downs of Weight Loss without Wellness

If you are reading this book you probably have been on at least two kinds of diets in your life. Chances are you have been on a lot more than two. Perhaps you are one of the 16 percent of all women who are continually on a diet. That is the category I was in. I used to tell people that I had been on a diet since age twelve.

Well, you and I are not alone. According to a government study in 1986, 32 million adult Americans are overweight and almost 16 million are severely overweight. Being overweight can often make you feel desperate about your life, and this desperate feeling encourages you to "try anything." A "try anything" attitude is what draws people to all of the various diets that are on the latest best-seller list at the bookstore. Unfortunately these diets, as you already know, do not work.

Statistics demonstrate that of the millions of people who go on diets every year and lose weight, only 3 percent keep the weight off. The other 97 percent lose the weight and then, bingo, put it right back on. Talk about desperation!

What is it about diets that keeps them from working? What makes the Wellness diet different from all the other diets out there? Well, simply put, this diet takes *work* whereas almost all the other diets promise something for nothing. Like almost everything else in life, if it is "something for nothing" it must be too good to be true. In the area of dieting, something for nothing *is* too good to be true.

WHY THE OTHER DIETS DO NOT WORK

One of the biggest reasons that other diets do not work is that they do not change the Fat Stat of your body. In fact, it is the Fat Stat which sabotages the diet. Here is how that sabotage happens.

Let us say you go on a diet that allows only 500 calories a day, and those calories can be obtained from any kind of food. Your body says "Whoa, what's going on?" and tries to stop you from losing weight by activating your Fat Stat. While you are on a restricted diet, your Fat Stat is trying to *preserve* your weight and not allowing it to go down. This causes your metabolic rate, the rate at which your body burns calories, to go down. If it goes down, then your body will need fewer calories to maintain weight. So it follows that if your body needs fewer calories to maintain weight, then even though you have restricted your calorie intake your body will actually need *fewer* calories. In other words you will not lose weight. Having slowed down your eating habits, your body slows down too. Imagine your body in slow motion. To hold onto its weight, your body's metabolism slows down to use fewer calories. If you were stranded on a desert island without food this might help preserve your health, but barring that situation, you are out of luck.

Of course, if you really restrict your caloric intake (with starvation, for example), or if you go on a limited calorie diet for a period of two or three weeks, you will lose weight. This will happen because your Fat Stat can maintain your weight for only a limited amount of time. If you continually consume fewer calories than your body expends, you will lose weight. But then what happens when you start to eat normally again? Your Fat Stat goes wild with excitement when it sees all that food. It tries to return your body to its previous weight and to retrieve all the weight you lost. It soaks up the extra calories (extra because you had been consuming so few) and zaps the weight back on.

The Fat Stat asked your body to conserve energy while you were dieting, so when you eat normally your body takes a while to adjust. During this adjustment period the body gains weight very rapidly because the Fat Stat is still busy conserving energy. Therefore, the normal caloric intake of 1500 will seem like 2000 or 2500 to your body and it will store those "extra" calories as fat. Remember, we evolved in a struggle for survival of the fittest. The fittest human being would be one who could survive during periods of drought and other natural disasters when food was unavailable. Therefore, the slowing down of metabolism for preservation of body weight was helpful in evolution and a positive attribute. However, it is not a positive attribute when you are trying to lose weight. Consequently, while it might have taken you a month to lose 5 pounds, it may take you only two weeks to gain the 5 pounds right back. Not only will you gain the 5 pounds back, but often, you will gain an *extra* pound or two as well.

As your Fat Stat is subjected over and over again to calorie restrictive weight loss diets, such as starvation or very low calorie diets, it works harder to maintain your weight. So the more diets you have been on, the harder the Fat Stat fights against you. The more the Fat Stat fights back, the harder it is to lose weight and the easier it is to gain that lost weight back, plus a few extra pounds along the way.

OTHER FACTORS IN THE DIETER'S DILEMMA

Another reason why low calorie or starvation diets don't work is also related to the Fat Stat. If you are eating less, and your body is burning less fuel, you tend to fcel tired and listless. Your activity level decreases, and this decrease will individually act to raise the Fat Stat. In other words, the Fat Stat functions to conserve your body's energy by making it more efficient. This will "protect" it against starvation. So while you are trying to lose the weight, your Fat Stat is trying to maintain your present weight. It all winds down to the number of calories your body needs. Again, this sequence of events will ultimately sabotage your attempt at weight loss.

When you are on a very low calorie or starvation diet, other things happen to your body. As you initially lose weight, the weight you lose is composed of more muscle tissue than fat tissue. So while the scale may drop, you are not really dropping fat—you are losing precious muscle. This does not occur if you lose weight more gradually and alter the Fat Stat as you go along.

Low calorie or starvation diets also affect your body's response to insulin. You are probably familiar with insulin in relation to someone who is a diabetic. Insulin is the hormone that helps the body store fat. A starvation or low calorie diet affects your body's response to this hormone, which causes increased fat storage. Because the Fat Stat is activated, your body is more sensitive to insulin. Insulin causes the body to store fat. When you are extra sensitive to insulin, fat is stored more easily. Again, this is an example of your body trying to protect itself by maintaining weight—exactly the opposite of what you want it to do.

Sometimes it is difficult to understand why it is so hard to lose weight in certain parts of your body. I am sure you have experienced weight loss in all the parts of your body you don't want to lose weight in. First your cheeks start to look hollow—a look that some of us like if we have high cheekbones, but also a look that some of us would rather not possess. Next your rings start to fall off your fingers. Then your breasts get smaller, and smaller, and smaller. All the while you are losing "weight" your thighs, belly, and hips remain their "larger than pleasing" size. In men, weight loss also begins in the cheeks and hands. It seems the last thing to start shrinking is the "spare tire" around the middle. Why, oh why?

Part of the explanation lies in the different types of fat cells in these areas. Because of their unique metabolism, the fat cells in the face, hands, and breasts are easily broken down and let go of their fat, shrinking rapidly. The fat cells in the thighs, hips, and belly hang onto their fat and only reluctantly give it up. So when you start losing weight, it first comes off from the cells that lose it the easiest—the fat cells in the face, hands, and breasts. To start losing weight in these problem areas you first need to deplete the stores of fat in the face, hands, and breasts. Only then will you start to lose in the other, more stubborn areas. If you lose weight more slowly, as you do with the Wellness Way to Weight Loss diet, the body tends to lose weight more evenly and from all areas at once. Early weight loss will still favor the hands, face, and breasts, but the difference isn't as dramatic as with rapid weight loss.

Similarly, if you gain weight back after you have lost it, the first areas to suck that weight up are the problem areas. Obviously this is a very difficult situation and another reason why drastically cutting back on calories does not work.

PROBLEMS WITH SOME OF THE CURRENT FAD DIETS

Most of the problems with the current fad diets are related to inadequate manipulation of the Fat Stat. If you don't alter the Fat Stat, it will continually work against you in weight loss and weight maintenance. However, individual diets have additional difficulties besides the Fat Stat problem, some of which are quite serious. A few of the most popular diets and their attendant problems are discussed below.

The Rice and Fruit Diet

Originally formulated for patients who had severe blood pressure problems and kidney disease, the rice and fruit diet is low in calories, fat, protein, salt, and cholesterol.

The problem with this diet, in addition to its being very low calorie with no modification of the Fat Stat, is that it is inherently unbalanced. Essentially the diet consists of two food groups—grain and fruit. With such a limitation on food groups, there is a real risk of inadequate intake of essential vitamins and minerals. In fact, in some major hospitals where the "rice diet" is used, the patients are monitored very closely and are given supplements to prevent vitamin and mineral deficiencies. Among the important vitamins and minerals lacking in this diet is calcium, which is an essential mineral for everyone, especially women. An inadequate calcium intake puts you at increased risk for developing brittle, easily breakable bones—a condition called *osteoporosis*—after you reach menopause. Breaking a hip after menopause can have disastrous consequences. Research has shown that half of all elderly people who break a hip die within one year of complications from the fracture.

The Diet That Rotates Foods

This diet rotates the calorie intake of dieters. Dieters consume low numbers of calories on a three- and four-day plan for the first week. This low calorie week is followed by a week of slightly higher calorie intake, which is then followed by another low calorie week. After the third week, the dieter gets a vacation from dieting. The length of this vacation is self-determined.

The potential difficulties with this diet are its low level of calories and inadequate manipulation of the Fat Stat. Additional problems are again related to the diet's lack of balance in partaking of all food groups. It is almost impossible to achieve balanced nutrition on the low level of calories that are recommended. Vitamin and mineral supplements are recommended to accompany this diet, but this is not enough to counteract the basic unbalanced nature of the diet.

The Diet That Claims to Make You Fit

This diet maintains that if you follow it you will lose weight permanently. It also maintains that calorie counting is not the best means of achieving weight loss. This diet states that lowering calorie intake won't affect weight loss unless you avoid food which is considered toxic or harmful to the body. The diet then directs you to avoid certain foods that it says are toxic. Also, this diet claims that human digestion functions in three 8-hour shifts during each 24-hour period. The diet is based on adjustments in food intake to accommodate these shifts. In addition, the diet claims that different food types should not be eaten together.

Again this diet has problems similar to others in that it is not well-balanced and can be very deficient in certain nutrients. The nutrients which are often deficient include Vitamin C, calcium, iron, zinc, and selenium. The claims of 8-hour shifts in digestion and the existence of "toxic" substances defined in the diet have questionable substantiation in the medical literature.

The Liquid Diets

Very popular with the American public, the liquid diets are those usually endorsed by television and sport celebrities. On liquid diets you substitute a liquid diet-food mixture for your meals. Some liquid diets require you to replace breakfast and lunch with the liquid and then eat a "normal" dinner. Other very low calorie liquid diets substitute all your meals for the liquid mixture. On these diets you may not eat any solid foods for weeks.

If you follow liquid diets you *will* lose weight. Although weight loss is more rapid on the very low calorie diets, both diets cause you to shed pounds. The problem is keeping the weight off. The weight loss is fairly easy while you are drinking the liquid because you don't have to make any choices about food consumption. You only choose between two things: drinking the liquid or going off the diet. Therefore, when you are following the liquid diet you aren't modifying your eating habits, and you aren't learning about healthy food choices and how to control your appetite.

Therefore, when you go off the liquids and start eating solid foods, your old habits are still with you. If you overate before, you will still overeat; if you ate a lot of fatty foods, you will still eat a lot of fatty foods. If you eat because you are stressed and not because you are hungry, this type of eating pattern will continue. In short, all the things that caused you to be overweight before you went on a diet will still be operating when you go off the diet. No education or habit changes will have occurred in the meantime. This is why the people who lose weight on these diets rarely keep the weight off.

FAD DIETS IN GENERAL

The diets described above are just a few of the many fad diets Americans have selected over the years in their desperate attempt to lose weight. I have selected these diets to illustrate some of the common problems that exist in almost all fad diets. As discussed above, these problems include inadequate manipulation of the Fat Stat, nutrient deficiencies, and, sometimes, outright misinformation.

First and foremost, any time you stay on a restricted calorie intake diet your Fat Stat causes your metabolic rate to slow down and you burn fewer and fewer calories. This makes it harder to lose weight. Without manipulation of the Fat Stat, weight loss will be very difficult to achieve and next to impossible to maintain.

The second problem, nutrient deficiencies, occurs because these diets are unbalanced and therefore contain inadequate nutrients such as vitamins and minerals, which are essential for healthy nutrition. Diets which lack vitamins and minerals are hazardous to your health. This is especially true for women in general and pregnant women in particular. Without adequate nutrient intake our bodies become deficient, resulting in weak bones; brittle hair and nails that grow slowly; dry, flaky, scaly skin; problems making hormones in the body and the brain; and interrupted bodily functions. In short, losing weight at the expense of vitamins and minerals is not a nutritionally good idea and can be very hazardous to your health.

A third problem with fad diets is that often they are based on nonmedical and/or unproven nutritional theories. Many times, authors of diet books use nutritional theories which are untested, or even later disproved.

If any of these diet books were as good as they claimed or really delivered an effective and permanent weight loss program, then every doctor in the country would be prescribing them. But unfortunately they don't work. Most diets promise something for nothing. But losing weight and keeping it off requires work—plain and simple.

WHAT IS DIFFERENT ABOUT THE WELLNESS WAY TO WEIGHT LOSS DIET?

The Wellness Way to Weight Loss diet works because of several different factors. First and foremost, eating the Wellness way ensures basic good nutrition. When you eat the Wellness way, you can be assured that you are providing your body with the vitamins and minerals it needs to function properly.

When you eat the Wellness way and consume fewer calories than your body requires to maintain weight, and you exercise a minimal amount as described in the chapter on exercise, then you can alter your Fat Stat. This alteration of the Fat Stat will allow you to lose weight and, at long last, keep it off permanently. Exercise is a necessary part of any permanent weight loss program. But exercise will not cure the deficiencies noted in the other diets described.

After following the Wellness Way to Weight Loss diet you will be educated about proper nutrition. Eating the Wellness way will become second nature. You will be relieved to escape the vicious cycle of dieting and losing and gaining and dieting again. You will be able to eat and feel full instead of feeling deprived. Finally, not only will you be maintaining your optimal weight but you will be protecting yourself against disease as well.

SOME SPECIFICS OF THE WELLNESS DIET AND WEIGHT LOSS

The Wellness Way to Weight Loss is made up of two principles—proper nutrition and proper exercise. Only these two principles *combined* can alter your Fat Stat.

Combining these two principles, you can work on the factors within your control that are contributing to your excess weight. These factors include your Fat Stat, inactivity, and food intake.

5

Why Do We Overeat?

The obvious answer to the question "Why do we eat?" is that we get hungry and we need food to survive. If this were the only stimulus for eating, none of us would have a weight problem. We have an appetite because this desire for food encourages us to eat, and eating is necessary for life. If we did not have an appetite, then we would have no stimulus to eat and we would die. The problem is that there are many other stimuli besides survival that arouse our appetite. These stimuli include psychological and environmental factors, and it is these additional factors that are primarily responsible for the problem of overeating. Here we will focus on the factors that contribute to our desire to overeat.

PSYCHOLOGICAL FACTORS

There are many psychological factors that contribute to overeating. Some can be a sign of an underlying depression whereas others are societal in nature. Whatever the reason for overeating, it must be uncovered if we are to reach and maintain an ideal body weight.

Stress

Stress is one of the most influential motivators of appetite. Often we eat in an attempt to alleviate stress. Food is a comfort. If you are nervous about your job, home life, or social life, eating seems to help you calm down. But think about it: when you are feeling stress, you are usually moving at a rapid rate of speed. Even if you aren't physically running around, your body is running at a higher rate of speed. When you are stressed, your heart rate, breathing rate, and blood pressure all are higher than normal. When you stop to eat, it is actually the experience of slowing down and stopping that has a tendency to calm you down—not necessarily the eating. Your heart rate and respiratory rate slow; you calm down. But your body only knows that it feels better once you stop and eat, and it can't differentiate the stopping from the eating. Therefore, your body associates the comfort derived from the stopping and eating to the act of eating. When you are stressed, your body subconsciously seeks comfort, and eating often provides this comfort. So when you are stressed you will often find yourself eating more in an unconscious attempt to comfort yourself by slowing down.

How do you know if you are experiencing stress? There are many clues and telltale signs of stress. The greater the number of these telltale signs you have, the more stress you are feeling. Some of the signs of stress are:

- Cold hands
- Eyestrain and frequent blinking
- Gritting of teeth

- Elevated blood pressure
- Shallow breathing
- Irritability
- Nervous jittering of knees
- Tapping of fingers
- Loss of sense of humor
- Loss of interest in sex
- Sleeping problems, whether you are unable to sleep or oversleep
- Upset or churning stomach
- Difficulty concentrating
- Drinking too much alcohol
- Feeling tense or anxious
- Feeling inadequate

Frequently patients come to see me complaining of tiredness and an upset, churning stomach. Most often, after examining them and questioning them about what is happening in their lives, it turns out that they are not afflicted with any dreaded disease. Rather, they are experiencing stress-related symptoms. Very often it is difficult to convince a patient that he or she is indeed stressed. The patient says, "I don't feel stressed" or "I can't think of anything that is stressing me." Then we usually go over the symptoms of stress listed above and frequently the patient will say, "Yes, I do experience some of those things, but I don't know why I am stressed." I usually reply that it is sometimes difficult to identify specific stressors. Often, a person experiencing stress will not have a major catastrophic event occurring such as a divorce or death, but will still feel stressed. You can be experiencing a combination of stressors—your job, traffic, children, your relationships—all of which can contribute to feelings of stress. These are examples of subtle stressors that can drive you to overeat just as much as the megastressors such as death, divorce, illness, and accidents. To overcome stress-induced eating, you must recognize and overcome your stress.

There are many methods of dealing with stress and its effects on your body. Exercise is a great method of stress reduction. When you exercise your mind is concentrating on the exercise rather than on your stress, whether consciously or subconsciously. This aids the body in its attempt to relax. The same principles apply to the way meditation and relaxation techniques relax the body. When you meditate you concentrate on an image. By concentrating on an image you cannot concentrate on your stressors, and your body automatically relaxes. Researchers have placed electrodes onto individuals' forehead muscles. When these individuals were stressed, their forehead muscles were tense. As they meditated, the tension in their forehead muscles gradually decreased until it reached a baseline level.

The stress reduction technique that I prescribe most frequently is the "tension relaxation technique." To use this method, all you need is a quiet space. This means that you tell your kids, roommate, husband, dogs, or anyone else not to disturb you until you come out of your space. Your space may be your bedroom, den, or even the bathroom. Sit in a comfortable chair with your arms and legs uncrossed. Shut your eyes and progressively tense and relax your muscles. Start with your facial muscles and move down your body—your neck muscles, shoulder muscles, arm muscles, stomach muscles, buttocks muscles, thigh muscles, calf muscles, and foot muscles. Tense these muscles for 10 seconds, then relax them for about 30 seconds. Don't be concerned about counting exactly 30 seconds or 10 seconds. If you get too concerned about the time or doing the technique exactly right, then you will stress yourself in the middle of your stress reduction exercise.

Practice this technique twice a day—it only takes about 10 minutes. You will notice almost immediately that when you emerge from your space you will feel more relaxed and centered than before you started. After a period of time, you will notice that the relaxed feeling lasts longer and longer. Eventually, if you find yourself in a stressful situation, you can relax your body by tensing your hand (clenching your fist) and then relaxing it. Your brain will be programmed to respond to tensing and relaxing muscles by relaxing your whole body. This is a fast stress reduction technique that is very useful in situations in which you can't go to a space and complete the whole tensing and relaxing series. This technique can be used while in the car, waiting at a light or while stopped in traffic, or while you are at work. Another quick relaxation technique is deep breathing. A few very deep breaths, slowly breathing in and out, have a remarkable calming effect.

Other methods to reduce stress involve taking a critical look at your life. For example, you might experience a lot less stress if you didn't have to work, but then you couldn't eat or clothe yourself because you wouldn't have any money. Try not to say "yes" to every request that is put to you. If you meet a problem, try to discuss it with your superior instead of bottling up your anger or frustration. Use this same technique at home with your loved ones. If you fail, tell yourself that you have failed and not that you are a failure. If you are late or stuck in traffic, take a moment to say to yourself, "I will not get there any faster by getting all worked up, and getting all worked up won't make the traffic go away." Try to control only those situations that are controllable.

Boredom

Bored individuals typically eat more than active individuals. Eating fills up time. Preparing food (which, of course, you sample during preparation) alleviates boredom. Attending parties because you have nothing else to do also contributes to overeating. To overcome eating due to boredom you must develop an alternative activity. Consider an exercise program. Another method which could help to combat boredom includes volunteering for activities. These can be community service activities or work-related activities. You may consider seeking a second job or going back to school.

Depression

One of the most common signs of depression is weight gain because individuals who are depressed frequently gain weight. If you are depressed, you have a tendency to gain weight for a number of different reasons.

The first reason for weight gain is similar to the reason that stressed individuals gain weight—food provides comfort. When you are depressed, as when you are stressed, you desire comfort and food answers part of this desire.

Another reason that you gain weight when you are depressed is because of your relative inactivity. When you are depressed you feel a remarkable lack of energy. It often seems to be a chore to just get out of bed. Because you have such a low energy level, you sit for longer periods of time and are generally much less physically active then you normally are. This decrease in activity means that your body needs fewer calories than usual to maintain weight. However, you usually eat more when you are depressed. So couple eating more with expending fewer calories because of your inactivity and you can see that you are a set-up to gain weight.

Emotional Starvation

If you are lonely, you will often eat because you feel emotionally starved. Many people eat as a substitute for the comfort and solace they are not getting from themselves or from a relationship. To overcome this eating habit you must comfort yourself in other ways besides eating food.

Environmental Stress

People tend to overeat when they are cold, a result of evolution. Our ancestors ate more when they were cold in order to add a layer of fat that would serve as protection. This was of great benefit to our ancestors when they lived in huts and igloos, but it doesn't help us in our insulated homes — it only helps us to be fat. Be aware of this tendency to overeat when it is cold. If you are aware of it, then you can attempt to fight it off. If you are not aware of it, then you won't fight it off—you will eat.

COPING WITH THE REASONS FOR OVEREATING

There are many methods of coping with the different causes of overeating. These methods may involve reading self-help books which talk about self-esteem and learning to love yourself. You might consider joining a support group or seeking psychological counseling. Any method of learning about yourself and what motivates your actions (including the action of eating) will help you to control the eating which you are using to satisfy yourself.

Whether it is reading books, joining a group, or undergoing individual counseling, the secret of fending off the stimulus to overeat is to look within yourself. The different methods of counseling will aid you in searching within yourself for the reasons that you are depressed, feel stressed, or are bored or lonely. Try helping yourself by reading or schedule an appointment with your doctor to discuss the matter. Often your doctor will recommend certain books or may even suggest that you seek therapy in a group or from a counselor. Once you gain insight as to why you are overeating, it usually is a little easier to say no to yourself by saying no to food. Certainly every little bit of understanding that you gain about yourself will help you on your quest for a Wellness life-style.

As you can see, there are many factors behind hunger which can increase our desire to eat. These factors must be identified and modified in our never-ending quest for Wellness. Of all the factors, stress is one of the biggest motivators of overeating. Each can be understood and dealt with successfully once you have committed yourself to a Wellness life-style.

6

Fiber

The Great Warrior in Weight Loss

Fiber is one of the most important foodstuffs in a Wellness diet. In fact, it is the cornerstone of a Wellness diet. It is astounding that, until recently, this group of foods, which has been around for such a long time, has gotten so little attention. Fiber was once much more common in the American diet than it is now. Over the years refined foods such as cakes and cookies have replaced many of the high fiber foods we used to enjoy, such as fruits, vegetables, whole grain breads, and cereals.

America shifted its attention back to fiber in the early 1970s, when evidence began surfacing that fiber lowered the incidence of certain diseases. Reports began to materialize linking diets high in fiber with a lowered rate of cancer of the bowel and other intestinal diseases such as hemorrhoids, hiatal hernia, gallstones, and appendicitis.

These diseases were very common among Americans and in other industrialized societies where the typical diet was low in fiber. Thus, interest in fiber was rekindled. Fiber is not only great as a preventative of disease but also is an essential part of a Wellness diet.

All fiber comes from plants. Foods which are high in naturally occurring carbohydrates are usually also high in fiber. We all know fiber as roughage or "bran."

Fiber is not a true nutrient because it is not completely digestible. Although you "eat" fiber, your body can't break it down completely to digest it. Fiber is a great Wellness and weight loss aid because even though you eat it, it is like getting some "free calories" because you don't absorb it. Fiber fills you up—not out. You can eat and feel full, but because part of what you eat is fiber, you will absorb fewer calories than when you eat the same amount of a fat or protein type of food.

Different types of fiber are digested differently by the body. The two basic types of fiber are soluble and insoluble. Soluble fiber foods are those which dissolve in water like the fiber in fruits. A type of soluble fiber is pectin. You may remember your mother or grandmother or even yourself using pectin in making jelly. Pectin was added to the pureed fruit, causing it to gel by holding the water in suspension. Another type of soluble fiber is in guar gum, which also helps to hold water in suspension. Pectin is a natural softener and can be found in such foods as apple peel and the skin citrus fruits—oranges, lemons, and grapefruit. Guar gum is commonly found in beans. Other soluble fibers are the fibers found in beans, carrots, and rolled oats, although these vegetables and grains contain insoluble fiber as well.

Insoluble fibers are those fibers which do not dissolve in water or in your body. Fibers that are insoluble are cellulose and psyllium. Cellulose fiber is found in bran, which is usually what most people think of in terms of fiber food. Psyllium is a type of fiber derived from a seed which originates in Asia Minor.

Because both psyllium and cellulose are insoluble, they are not dissolved at all in your body. Rather than being natural softeners like pectin and guar gum, they are bulk producers—that is, they make your stool more bulky, which really is a sign of good health.

The most common source of fiber in the average diet comes from cereals and fruits. The average diet contains only 15 grams of fiber. For Wellness and weight loss, 25 to 30 grams of fiber are recommended. In addition, with increased importance being placed on fiber, extra fiber, like pectin and cellulose, is being added to food products to increase the total fiber content. Breads and cereals are examples of food products that sometimes contain extra added fiber.

FIBER AND WEIGHT LOSS

Fiber is an amazing food with many remarkable properties: it is your best warrior in the weight loss battle. Fiber has remarkable properties to aid in weight loss and weight control. High fiber foods, whether soluble or insoluble, are bulky foods. Fiber acts like a sponge to soak up water. When you add this to bulk, fiber foods take up more room in your stomach. Therefore, you feel full more quickly with a lesser amount of food. The more fiber your diet contains, the fewer calories you are likely to consume.

Foods that are high in fiber take longer to chew. Think about how long it takes to chew broccoli or popcorn. This extra chewing time allows your stomach to "catch up" with your brain, making you feel full sooner than when you rapidly eat other foods. All of the chewing helps you feel like you have eaten more then you really have.

Foods that are fiber-rich reduce the number of calories your body absorbs from the food you eat. This occurs because the fiber causes the food to pass through the bowel at a more rapid rate. Due to this quick passage, the bowel cannot absorb the same number of calories from the food substance as it would if things moved more slowly. Some studies have shown that your body is less efficient in digesting high fiber foods, and so some calories you would otherwise have absorbed are passed through your body and not to your body.

HOW TO ADD FIBER TO YOUR DIET

Now that I have extolled the virtues of fiber, let us get down to the basics of how to add the proper amount of fiber to your diet. First, before you drastically change your diet to include high amounts of fiber, I recommend that you discuss the changes with your doctor. This is especially true if you have any type of bowel disease that may lead to a blockage of your bowel. This can occur after you have had surgery in your abdomen like a hysterectomy. Also, check with your doctor first if he or she has already recommended a special diet for you.

Fiber has the unique property of binding or grabbing food substances that are in the bowel at the same time. This binding or grabbing causes the foodstuff, whether it is fat or another nutrient, to pass through the body without being absorbed. In addition, since fiber is so good at carrying things through the bowel and binding substances like fats, fiber can also bind other substances like vital nutrients. It is good when fiber binds fats and sugars and they are not absorbed or when it binds possible cancer-causing chemicals. However, when fiber binds nutrients or minerals, you run the risk of becoming deficient in these nutrients. This is not usually a problem if you follow the well-balanced Wellness diet I recommend, since you will be consuming enough nutrients to make up for any which are lost through your body. However, if you do not follow a well-balanced diet, you run the risk of becoming nutrient and vitamin deficient. One of these minerals is calcium, and, as we noted earlier, women in particular must ensure that they have adequate calcium intake to stave off osteoporosis in their menopausal years.

SOME POSSIBLE PROBLEMS

The most common problem with increasing the amount of fiber in your diet is a matter of social embarrassment—increased intestinal gas. Many times after commenting on the virtues of fiber to one of my patients, the patient will return later saying, in an embarrassed manner, "Doc, I feel better on this high fiber diet and I'm losing weight, but my family is really having a hard time with all this gas I'm producing!"

This increase in gas is usually only temporary. The bacteria in your bowels interact with the fiber substances you ingest and cause them to ferment, producing gas. The problem is greatly reduced if you increase the amount of fiber in your diet in a gradual way.

Finally, if you add fiber to your diet and don't drink more water with it, you can paradoxically give yourself a bout of constipation. This occurs because the fiber, whether soluble or insoluble, absorbs water, and unless you drink extra water it can dry your stool substance and cause you to become constipated. To avoid this problem, drink at least eight 8-ounce glasses of water a day. Seltzer and sugar-free diet sodas are alternatives to water, but water is still the ideal fluid.

RECOMMENDATIONS FOR FIBER

There is no absolute recommendation as to just how much fiber in the diet is enough. However, I usually have my patients set a goal of 30 grams for their total daily fiber intake. It is essential that this fiber come from a variety of foods and that the 30-gram total be approached gradually. Start adding fiber to your diet slowly. The usual rule of thumb is to add only 5 grams every two weeks until the 30-gram level is reached. Start by adding a serving of bran or whole grain with each meal in the form of cereal, bread, crackers, muffins, or rice. Then gradually add more vegetables and fruits and more bran and whole grain until you reach 30 milligrams of fiber.

To increase your fiber intake choose carbohydrates packaged in their natural fibrous coatings. Use brown rice instead of white, whole grain flour instead of white flour, and whole grain crackers, breads, and cereals. In a similar way, choose vegetables with edible skins and seeds such as squash and tomatoes. These choices enable you to ingest both soluble and insoluble fibers.

The vegetables can be fresh, frozen, or canned. Rinsing the canned vegetables will remove unwanted and unneeded salt, which can be problematic if you have high blood pressure. Also, choose fruits with edible skins and seeds. The fruits can be raw or canned in their own juice, and I would suggest eating more whole fruits rather than fruit juices.

Dried beans and dried peas may be hard to digest at first, so start with the easily digested kinds such as lentils, split peas, and lima beans. If you tolerate these well without too much gas, then advance to other kinds such as navy, pinto, kidney, and black beans.

Use more grains such as rice and bran in your meal plan. Popcorn is a great source of fiber as well as a low calorie and nutritious snack—without the butter and salt, of course. Watch your calorie intake!

Turn low fiber foods into high fiber foods. When a recipe calls for bread crumbs, use bran. Use bran in meatloaf and casseroles. Use whole wheat noodles instead of egg noodles. Sprinkle psyllium seed or husks on toast and sandwiches. Eat bran cereal instead of low fiber cereals.

In addition to all their benefits, high fiber foods do have calories, although usually not as many as other foods. In the Wellness Way to Weight Loss diet this concept is addressed in detail. The recommended calories include those recommended for fiber. If you eat extra calories by adding high fiber foods to your daily food intake, you won't lose weight, you will gain it. Instead, substitute fiber foods for other foods. The Wellness Way to Weight Loss diet incorporates high fiber foods into your daily caloric intake. Follow your Wellness diet and reduce your intake of high fat, high calorie foods while simultaneously increasing your high fiber foods.

TIPS TO INCREASE THE FIBER IN YOUR DIET

Some quick and simple tips on increasing your total daily fiber intake are as follows:

- Eat a variety of fiber-rich foods.
- Increase your intake of whole-grain breads and cereals.
- Eat more vegetables—at least two servings each of raw or cooked vegetables each day, with the skins.

- Concentrate on high fiber vegetables: lentils, split peas, kidney beans, and other beans.
- Have a bowl of bran cereal at least three times a week.
- Leave the skins on potatoes; this adds to their fiber content.
- Use more vegetarian-type meat substitutes such as beans, peas, nuts, and seeds.
- Use more fruits for dessert and snacks.
- Eat all kinds of fruit and leave on the skin.
- Eat brown and wild rice instead of white rice.

REMEMBER: Watch the calories. Just because you are eating fiber does not mean the food is noncaloric. When you eat extra calories by increasing your fiber intake, those calories must be substituted calories. Substitution is based on the exchange system, which is discussed in the diet chapter. But also remember that the more fiber you eat, the less fat and calories you absorb, so you are in a win–win situation!

7

Fiber and Disease

Fiber is a great fighter against a multitude of diseases. This fighting ability is due to the remarkable properties of fiber we just examined. Now I will key in on some of the many diseases that fiber helps prevent and that fiber can actually help treat.

FIBER AND BOWEL DISEASE

Fiber is a great chemical-free way to decrease your chance of acquiring bowel disease. Fiber is also a chemical-free way to control a bowel disease you may already have. The type of fiber found in bran and other whole grains is especially beneficial in preventing and aiding in the treatment of bowel disease. Some of these diseases are irritable bowel syndrome (also known as colitis), diverticulitis, hemorrhoids, and constipation.

Irritable Bowel Syndrome

Irritable bowel syndrome is a very common disease in the United States. Not a day goes by without someone walking into my office with irritable bowel syndrome. The symptoms of irritable bowel syndrome include crampy abdominal pain, increased gas, and alternating diarrhea and constipation. The symptoms can and usually are made far worse with increased stress. Irritable bowel syndrome is a benign condition in that it is not lethal, but it does cause many people to be quite miserable. Irritable bowel syndrome can really affect the quality of your life. It can, however, be controlled with a Wellness diet that is high in fiber. The fiber acts to calm the bowel, and persons affected by irritable bowel syndrome can then eat foods such as fruits and vegetables that ordinarily would upset them.

Diverticulitis

Diverticulitis is also a common disease in the United States, especially in people over the age of fifty. Diverticula are outpouchings of the bowel wall which are thought to develop because of increased pressure and wear and tear on the bowel wall. If one of these outpouchings becomes plugged, infection can occur, and with infection comes pain. The pain usually arises in the left lower side of the abdomen. A complication of diverticulitis, which can be fatal, is bowel rupture. Bowel rupture occurs when the diverticulum (the plugged-up pouch) becomes more and more full as a result of the build-up of material resulting from the infection. Finally, like a balloon, it can rupture, causing the contents of the bowel to spill out into the abdominal cavity. As you can imagine, bowel contents are full of germs, and it is the spread of these germs into the abdomen which can be fatal. So if your chances of developing diverticulitis can be lowered or eliminated, do it!

Diverticulitis is almost unheard of in populations which

routinely follow a Wellness diet high in fiber. Therefore, the culprits are diets high in refined foods and low in fiber. In the past, the treatment for diverticulosis, the state of having diverticula which are not inflamed, was to follow a diet which contained no seeds or roughage such as peanuts and popcorn. It was believed that these foodstuffs would plug up the diverticula, which would become inflamed, causing diverticulitis. However, the current treatment is to follow a Wellness diet high in fiber. Fiber's property of moving stuff quickly through the bowel keeps the other foodstuffs from plugging anything up and also decreases the pressure in the bowel. So eating rather than avoiding fiber helps in fighting diverticula.

Hemorrhoids

Almost everyone is familiar with hemorrhoids. They form due to increased pressure in the large bowel, especially in the rectum, which is the end of the large bowel. Hemorrhoids can itch and can be very painful. They can also bleed. Hemorrhoids are very common during pregnancy and in overweight people.

There are two kinds of hemorrhoids, internal and external. Both are caused by the same problem—increased pressure in the rectum. This increased pressure causes outpouching in the veins of the rectum, and these outpouchings are the hemorrhoids. A Wellness diet high in fiber decreases the pressure in the bowel. When the pressure is decreased hemorrhoids can disappear. This is a painless cure for hemorrhoids. Many times surgeons will recommend surgical removal or freezing of hemorrhoids. Lasers are now also being used to treat hemorrhoids. While these procedures work, they all can be very painful. In addition, if pressure in your rectum is still there after the hemorrhoids are removed, they will just recur and all the pain you underwent having them removed will have been in vain. Thus, following a Wellness diet will not only control or cure hemorrhoids but will also prevent them from ever occurring.

Constipation

As with hemorrhoids, almost everyone is familiar with constipation. Very often I see patients in my office whose primary complaint is constipation. Often, they have been suffering for years with the problem but are too embarrassed or consider it too small a problem to mention it to a physician. Children in my practice are brought in by their parents who say they are constipated. They are constipated because they eat refined sugars (cakes, brownies, and the like) and get almost no fiber.

Following a Wellness, high fiber diet will all but guarantee that you will never again suffer from constipation.

Fiber absorbs water. When fiber passes into the large bowel it increases the softness of the stool. Fiber also adds bulk to the stool, which makes it lighter. Thus, the stool passes through much more easily and without straining. Therefore, if you do not strain, you will have a marked reduction in hemorrhoids and be completely free from constipation.

FIBER AND CANCER

In addition to these benign bowel conditions, a Wellness diet high in fiber can also decrease your chance of contracting cancer of the bowel. Colon cancer (cancer of the large bowel) is the second most common cancer in the United States. There are many theories on why bowel cancer develops, some of which include increased pressure in the large bowel, increased fats in the diet, and decreased transit time of the bowel contents (the time it takes for the contents of the bowel to pass through).

As we have noted, fiber decreases the pressure in the large bowel by making the stool softer and adding bulk to it. This then decreases the risk of developing cancer of the large bowel. Fiber also decreases the absorption of fats from the foodstuffs in the bowel contents. This will be discussed in greater detail in Chapter 9, but suffice it to say that this fat absorption is another risk of developing cancer of the bowel that eating a diet high in fiber helps eliminate.

Also, as we have noted, fiber decreases the bowel transit time. One theory of bowel cancer development is that cancer-causing agents in the foods we eat sit against the lining of the large bowel. By speeding the foodstuffs through the large bowel, fiber decreases the time the harmful agents have to act. Consequently, the chance of developing cancer from these agents is decreased. As you can see, fiber is a significant component in the fight against cancer.

Risks of developing other types of cancer are also decreased by eating a Wellness diet. The risk of developing cancer of the breast, prostate, stomach, and uterus are increased by a diet high in fats and decreased by a diet high in fiber and low in fat. Again, this is due to fiber's almost miraculous ability to decrease absorption of fats. Fat itself has many harmful effects, one of which is to increase your chance of developing these types of cancer. The less fat you absorb, the less harm it can cause you. Therefore, increasing your fiber intake decreases your risk of breast and prostate cancer.

FIBER AND HEART DISEASE

If all this were not enough, fiber also decreases your risk of developing heart disease. Heart disease is affected by consuming a diet that is high in fat. Fiber, as we have seen, decreases the absorption of fat and thus decreases the risks of developing heart disease and stroke. The American Heart Association recommends a high fiber/low fat diet. Fiber binds up some of the fat you eat and helps keep your body from absorbing it. Also, fiber decreases the recirculation of bile resins, which are a chemical that the liver secretes into the intestine. The bile resins are absorbed back into the system and then the liver changes them into cholesterol in the bloodstream. As you know, high cholesterol is associated with a high incidence of heart disease.

Cholesterol causes heart disease by forming plaques along the walls of blood vessels. If these plaques become large enough, they can block the circulation to the heart muscle. When the circulation is blocked, a heart attack occurs. There have been many studies which correlate fat intake with elevated cholesterol in the blood and subsequent development of heart disease. Therefore, if a high fiber diet decreases your intake of fat, why not eat a high fiber diet and decrease your chance of heart attack and cancer and lose weight at the same time!

If your diet is high in fiber, you generally do not eat as many high fat foods. So the total amount of fat you consume goes down, further aiding your body in combating heart disease.

The fibers such as those contained in raw fruits and vegetables are especially helpful in reducing the risk of heart disease. This is also true of the type of fiber found in rolled oats, oatmeal, and carrots. Oat bran has become very popular recently. Some studies have shown that diets high in oat bran decrease your chance of heart disease more than diets high in other types of fiber.

FIBER AND DIABETES

Diabetes mellitus is a disorder of the body's ability to regulate the level of sugar in the blood. The problem with high blood sugar is that it causes changes in the arteries and veins, hastening the chance of developing heart disease and stroke. Diabetes also damages the kidneys, the arteries, and the veins of the eyes, which can result in kidney failure and blindness.

Following a Wellness diet, which includes high fiber, can greatly improve the regulation of the level of sugar in your blood, thus reducing the sugar's damaging effects. A high fiber diet helps dilute the sugar you eat. Fiber also decreases how much sugar you can absorb; thus, your body isn't subjected to the damaging effects of high sugar. Studies have demonstrated fiber's profound effect on how the body absorbs sugar. One such study measured the blood sugar of diabetic patients, some of whom drank pectin-free (fiber-free) apple juice and others who ate the same number of calories of unpeeled apples (a high fiber food). Those that drank the juice had a high rise in their blood sugar while those who ate the apples had less of a rise. So you can see that fiber is a great aid in fighting diabetes and all of its medical complications because fiber aids the body in keeping the sugar at normal levels, not the high damaging levels.

Fiber is a wondrous food. It has remarkable properties which aid in fighting diseases such as cancer, heart attacks, and strokes.

8

Carbohydrates

The Good, the Bad, the Unnecessary

Carbohydrates have long gotten a bad press as "fattening foods." Remember all the diets in which you *couldn't* eat bread, potatoes, or pasta? Those diets were wrong. They were based on doctors' and nutritionists' claims that the starches found in carbohydrates made you fat. Starches were singled out as the culprit in obesity. In retrospect there is little evidence in the nutrition literature proving that starches and carbohydrates are deadly for the dieter. On the Wellness Way to Weight Loss diet, carbohydrates are a great ally in the battle to lose weight.

Why? Because carbohydrates provide energy for your body. Many carbohydrate foods contain fiber, so they aid in weight loss and maintenance based on the principles discussed in Chapter 6. However, in addition to those mechanisms, carbohydrate foods help weight loss in another way. Your body must use more energy to process or metabolize the carbohydrate foods than it would to process fat- or protein-rich foods. Through expending this extra energy, your body retains less of the food to be stored as extra weight.

For example, if you eat 100 calories of a carbohydrate food, your body uses 23 of those calories to process the food into a form it can use. Only 77 calories are available to be stored as fat. Compare this to eating 100 calories of fat. Your body uses only 3 calories in processing and stores 97 calories as fat. So with carbohydrates you are way ahead in the race against calories that are left over to be stored as fat. It becomes obvious that carbohydrates are another big ally in your endeavor to lose weight. Isn't it wonderful that the foods you love—spaghetti, pizza (without a lot of cheese), baked potatoes—are also foods that you can enjoy and that will help you lose weight and stay well? These foods are all high in carbohydrates and used to be forbidden foods on any diet. Now they are foods you can eat in plentiful amounts. Of course, the sauces, creams, and cheeses that are usually eaten with these high carbohydrate foods must be modified. No matter how good the carbohydrate, if a high fat cheese or high fat meat sauce is piled on top of it, the benefits of the carbohydrate will be lost against the fat content of the other foods.

High fiber foods are carbohydrate foods and are our weight-loss allies. There are many other types of carbohydrate foods, and they may or may not contain fiber. These foods can be divided into two types—simple and complex.

Sugars are simple carbohydrates and, in general, should be avoided. Table sugar is a good example of a simple carbohydrate. Simple carbohydrates are found in foods commonly considered desserts. Foods containing simple carbohydrates are high in sugar and include candy, cakes, pies, soft drinks, and ice cream. Usually the foods that are high in sugars are also high in fats—two reasons such food should be avoided. For example, a candy bar is composed of a high amount of sugar and the chocolate or caramel part of it is very high in fat. A lot of sugar, butter, lard, and flour are used to make pies, and heavy cream is an ingredient found in ice cream. In general, these dessert foods are almost always very high in fats as well as sugars and are not a part of a Wellness diet.

Complex carbohydrates are found in grains; the stems, leaves, and roots of vegetables; and in fruits. Examples of complex carbohydrate foods are potatoes, pasta, beans, and rice.

Simple and complex carbohydrates are defined by their chemical structure. Simple carbohydrates are simple sugars and have simple chemical structures whereas complex carbohydrates are complex sugars with complex structures.

Studies have shown that diets high in sugar promote weight gain. In fact, one study used two groups of rats to demonstrate the effects of sugar on weight gain: one group was fed chow food (a high fiber, high carbohydrate, low sugar food) while the other received only pure sugar. While the actual caloric intake was the same, the group eating the sugar gained weight. These test results further support the reasoning that "fattening" sugars will subvert you in your weight loss efforts and should be avoided. Eating complex carbohydrates, on the other hand, will encourage weight loss and promote general good health.

CARBOHYDRATES AND THE WELLNESS WAY TO WEIGHT LOSS

In 1920, the doctor's recommendation for the typical "good" American diet was to incorporate carbohydrates as only 20 percent of your diet. Again, this recommendation was founded on the hypothesis that carbohydrates were fattening foods, a hypothesis that really had no basis in fact. Now, the recommendations are that carbohydrate foods should make up 50 to 60 percent of your diet.

What Kind of Carbohydrates Should You Eat?

As we have seen earlier, simple sugars should be avoided. These foods are absorbed very rapidly by the body and, therefore, increase the level of sugar in the bloodstream. This sugar has the potential to be "grabbed" quickly by the body and later converted to fat stores. Complex carbohydrates, on the other hand, are absorbed more slowly and do not cause the blood sugar to peak as high; thus, those complex carbohydrates reduce the amount of sugar available to be stored by your body as fat.

Complex carbohydrates, because they are often high in fiber, also help you feel full more quickly then fatty and high protein foods do. Examples of complex carbohydrate foods that are also high in fiber are bran cereal and broccoli. Both contain high amounts of fiber and both are 100 percent carbohydrate. Therefore, when you eat these foods you are doing yourself a double favor.

Keep simple sugars to a minimum in your diet. Avoid table sugar, honey, candy bars, and corn syrup and sweet desserts like cakes, pies, and puddings. Natural sugars, like honey, are not any better for you than regular table sugar and should be avoided as well.

Concentrate on eating complex carbohydrates. Excellent sources of complex carbohydrates include grains such as wheat, rice, barley, and oats. Other sources are peas and various kinds of beans. Root vegetables like potatoes (sweet and white), turnips, and carrots are easily obtainable complex carbohydrates. The Wellness Way to Weight Loss diet endorses eating more pasta, whole grain breads, and fresh vegetables.

You might ask what kind of sauces should top such complex carbohydrates as pizza dough, pasta, and potatoes. The answer is to use low fat toppings. For pasta, use meatless tomato sauces and vegetable sauces — without the cream. For potatoes, use low calorie liquid margarine or, better yet, low calorie salad dressings. Pizza dough can be topped with tomato sauces and vegetables. There are many different ways to dress up carbohydrate foods which are exciting and interesting. Many of these recipes can be found in Chapter 13.

Both simple and complex carbohydrates can be refined. That means that they are processed from their natural state and added to other foods which do not naturally contain them. For example, table sugars and fructose are both simple sugars or carbohydrates which are added to the flour used in making cakes and pies. Another example is the addition of simple sugars to canned beans, fruits, yogurt, and peanut butter. Read the labels on packaged foods to identify hidden sugars. If sugar, corn sweeteners, or fructose are present, that food is said to be refined. To be refined is only to have simple sugars along as extra baggage. You are better off avoiding this extra baggage if at all possible, because it is not needed.

In general, your Wellness diet avoids refined or processed carbohydrate foods because they contain empty calories. These empty calories add to your total calorie intake and, thus, either add extra pounds or simply hinder your ability to lose weight quickly. Stick to naturally occurring complex carbohydrates.

The Wellness Way to Weight Loss diet contains complex, unrefined carbohydrates, and if you follow it closely you can protect yourself against eating hidden calories. While you are following the diet, you will be learning about the "good" carbohydrates and will begin to recognize the types of foods that are wise to avoid.

Carbohydrates are the cornerstone of a Wellness diet. They contain fiber and are the main source of the body's fuel. Rather than being the dieter's enemy, as once was thought, they are the dieter's greatest ally.

9

Fats

The Delicious but Dangerous Foods

WELLNESS AND FATS

A Wellness diet is as low in fats as much as it is high in fiber. Fats are a concentrated source of energy for your body and a necessary part of your diet. It is important, however, to know what kind of fat is good for you, what kind of fat is bad for you, what kind of fat you are now eating, and how much fat you should be eating.

To determine the good fats from the bad is not too difficult. Good fats are polyunsaturated and bad fats are saturated. A simple way to recognize a saturated fat, and thus a bad fat, is by asking yourself the following question: "Will this fat get hard if it is cooled?"

Animal fats obviously do get hard when cooled, as do butter, margarine, and some heavy creams. Other saturated and therefore bad fats do not fit this rule and have to be individually remembered. These are the fats in oils such as palm and coconut oil. Polyunsaturated fats, the good fats, always stay in a liquid form when cooled. Some examples are vegetable, safflower, sunflower, and corn oils. These are the good fats, which you can consume without too much worry. Still, as with any fat, you have to be careful of how much good fat you eat as part of your total daily diet.

SOME FATS ARE NECESSARY

Fats are a necessary part of your diet. They are the source of essential fatty acids, without which your body cannot make the fat it needs in certain areas such as the brain and spinal cord. The brain and spinal cord, both part of the nervous system, are primarily made up of fat. Dietary fats are also necessary for the transport of vitamins into your body and across the membranes of the cell walls. Fats form a "shell" around certain vitamins such as Vitamin A. Without such fat shells around them, some vitamins would just pass through your body. Similar fat shells are necessary for the microscopic transport of enzymes through the cell walls in your body. Enzymes act as catalysts for your metabolism. So fats are necessary, but only in limited amounts and only in the unsaturated form.

WHY DO WE LIKE FATS?

Basically, fats make food taste better. They add aroma, flavor, and texture to foods. Think about the smell of bacon frying or the flavor and texture of ice cream. These sensations all depend on the fat content of these foods. Fats also give you the satisfaction of feeling full because fats take longer to move through the stomach and intestinal system, which creates the sensation of fullness.

FATS MAKE YOU FAT

Of all the foodstuffs we consume, fat is the most fattening. Fat has more than two times as many calories per ounce than either protein or carbohydrates. Unfortunately, the average American diet consists of more than 40 percent fat—the equivalent of one stick of butter a day! Obviously, one of the first places to start in a Wellness diet, especially a Wellness diet to control your total weight, is to lower your fat intake.

Fats make you fat. Many studies have demonstrated that the proportion of daily calories which come from fats, rather than the number of calories you ingest, directly affects the degree of obesity.

Such studies also suggest why there are so many more overweight Americans now than at the turn of the century. Back then, the average American was eating 30 percent less total fat than is consumed today. Fat intake has been associated with higher standards of living, which have improved since the turn of the century. The higher the standard of living the more often meat is consumed, and meat is very high in fat. At the turn of the century carbohydrates such as potatoes and pasta were eaten in much greater proportion than meat. This resulted in a diet higher in carbohydrates and 30 percent lower in fat than today's average diet.

A smaller portion of high fat food often contains the same or even a greater number of calories than a larger portion of low fat food. Ounce for ounce, fat has more than double the calories than protein or carbohydrates. Two skinless chicken breasts about 3 ounces each are lower in fat and have fewer calories than a single lamb or pork chop (about 5 ounces).

But fats don't just increase your weight. They also lower your supply of nutrients. The more fat a food contains, the fewer nutrients it has in comparison with a low fat food of the same serving size. A doughnut, a high fat food, contains fewer vitamins and minerals than the same number of calories in a serving of a carbohydrate or protein.

One plain doughnut has as many calories as four slices of bread with 4 teaspoons of jam—about 400 calories. But in the doughnut, half of the calories come from fat, whereas only 10 percent of the calories in the bread and jam are from fat. The bread has significantly more nutrients than the doughnut. The body is much more efficient when converting dietary fat into body fat than it is when converting dietary carbohydrates, protein, and fiber into body fat. Therefore, the doughnut, even though it has the same number of calories as the bread and jam, is more fattening.

Sometimes it is difficult to identify the amount of fat you consume on a daily basis. Because it is hidden in many foods, you do not always realize when you are eating fat. Hidden fats can be found in foods like popcorn, cheese, and fried chicken. As an example consider french fries. French fries are made from potatoes which are high complex carbohydrate foods that you should try to include in your diet as often as possible. But when french fries are deep fried in oil, they soak up the fat like a sponge. Therefore, although you're eating a good food—potatoes—the fat hidden in them is fat that should be avoided in your diet. Moreover, frozen french fries are often treated with fattening oils before you even open the bag.

Another way fats are hidden in the foods we eat is through labels which may be misleading. Foods advertised as "low cholesterol" or "cholesterol-free" may still be loaded with fat.

Cholesterol is only one type of fat, and a cholesterol-free food may contain the other types of fat. An example would be peanut butter, which has no cholesterol but is 70 to 80 percent fat. Read the labels on foods and choose foods that are low in fat, not just low in cholesterol.

Fats are especially common in prepared foods. These foods are convenient to pop in the microwave oven but contain many hidden fats. Microwave popcorn at first seems like a good high fiber food. But most microwave popcorns are loaded with coconut or palm oil, which are highly saturated fats—fats you don't want or need.

However, once you have committed to memory the Wellness diet lists in this book, you will know where fats are hidden. No longer will you consume unknown amounts of fat and calories which add to your total weight gain. This knowledge alone will dramatically help you in your total Wellness plan of losing and maintaining your ideal weight. The tables found in the book and the recipes offered will help you become very familiar with high fat foods, medium fat foods, and low fat foods.

To determine how much fat a food contains simply read the label. The FDA requires that foodstuffs be labeled accurately. The label must specifically state how many grams of fat are contained in the product. To monitor your fat intake become a label fat reader. Don't be fooled by an oil labeled as "hydrogenated." Hydrogenated means hydrogen atoms were added to the fat, thus making it more saturated. A hydrogenated oil is therefore highly saturated and should be avoided whenever possible. There are many oils that are not hydrogenated and are unsaturated, such as safflower and sunflower oil. Try to use these oils instead of a hydrogenated oil.

If the food is something like fruit or bakery items, it may not have a label. If there is no label, look the food up in the table in Chapter 17.

HOW TO GET THE FAT OUT OF YOUR DIET

Your Wellness diet should contain 50 percent carbohydrates, 30 percent fat, and 20 percent protein. In Chapter 13, you will be given specific guidelines on how to ensure that your daily food intake conforms to these recommendations. But you can calculate how much fat is in your current diet by using the following formula:

> Read the label to determine how many grams of fat are in each serving of what you are eating. Each gram of fat contains nine calories. Multiply the grams by nine, the total of which equals the number of calories from fat. Then divide this number by the total number of calories, and you will have the percentage of fat calories in the food. For example, a cup of bran cereal contains 120 calories and 1 gram of fat. 1 (gram) × 9 = 9; 9 divided by 120 (calories) = .075; .075 × 100 = 7.5 percent.

Most of the fat you consume should be the unsaturated type. Again, a simple way to reduce the saturated fat you eat is to ask a single question about it: "Does this fat get hard?" If the answer is yes, it is a fat that you should avoid. Trim all of the fat off meats and skin chicken and turkey. These are animal fats and can be avoided simply by removing them. These are the fats that will make you fat and will increase your chances of developing all the problems associated with a high fat diet.

There are a number of simple guidelines to follow which will help get the fat out of your diet. To start, you can decrease or omit butter, margarine, mayonnaise, and cheese spreads from all the sandwiches and breads that you eat. You may be surprised at the lighter, different taste you will notice when it is not hidden by all that unhealthy fat.

Don't be fooled by salad dressings. You might think you are doing yourself a big favor by eating a salad, but if you load the salad with a lot of fatty salad dressing, you are doing more harm than good. Blue cheese salad dressing is one of the worst offenders; thousand-island-type dressings and high oil Italians are also very high in fat. Lemon juice, vinegar with just a little oil—say 1 teaspoon of oil for every 4 to 5 teaspoons of vinegar or lemon juice—and diet dressings are pleasant alternatives to top your salad.

Another way to cut down on fat is to avoid topping your vegetables with butter or margarine. Dipping your raw vegetables in a fatty dip also adds to the total fat in your diet. If you must have a buttery taste on your cooked vegetables, there are butter substitutes available that contain very little fat or fewer calories. These can be sprinkled on the hot vegetables to give them that buttery taste without the fat. Plain low fat yogurt with seasonings also can be a way to top your vegetables with a tasty surprise.

Change the way you prepare your food. Deep frying food dramatically increases the amount of fat in a food. As discussed, potatoes contain no fat but you can wring the fat out of french fries. Vegetables, meats, fish, and almost all food can be broiled, baked, or sauteed in a small amount of unsaturated oil, which can really drop the fat content. These types of cooking methods add much less fat to the food than frying them. Microwaving a food doesn't add to its fat content, and sauteeing in a Teflon-coated pan can decrease or eliminate the amount of oil necessary for cooking. Adding spices is a calorie-free way to enhance the taste of food.

When you bread food, you automatically increase its fat content. Most breaded food is high in fat because it contains not only the natural fat of the food, i.e., meat, but also the fat that makes the breading stick. Typically, breading is made with bread crumbs and oil or bread crumbs and egg. Both the egg and the oil are high fat foods. In addition, breading increases the amount of fat that a food will absorb while it is cooking. The breading soaks up as much fat as possible to coat the food and thereby adds to its fat content.

Because most meats are high fat foods, cutting down on your fat intake will mean eating less meat. This can be done by eating more meatless meals and by reducing the portions of the meat you do eat. You can do this by using meat as an addition to a dish rather than using it as a dish by itself. For example, the same 4-ounce serving used for a single serving of beef can be used for four servings of beef with peppers on top of rice.

Also, try to consume meats that are naturally lower in fat. Such meats include skinless chicken, turkey, fish, veal, and lean cuts of beef.

RECIPES

When you are cooking from recipes, use less fat than the recipe calls for. Reducing the amount of oil by half usually does not affect the taste and texture of most foods like bread, muffins, biscuits, sauces, and salad dressings.

Dairy Products

Dairy products in general are high in fat and thus the amount that you eat should be lowered. These include cheese, whole milk, and cream. You can adjust to the taste of skim or 1 percent milk and low fat cottage cheese. Low fat cheeses, such as Neufchatel and farmer's cheese, are now commonly available. Also, low fat yogurt has all the taste of yogurt but much less fat. In recipes, use whipped cottage cheese instead of sour cream and skim instead of whole milk.

Meats

Beef and pork are high fat meats. Especially high in fat are the marbleized cuts of beef. If you can see a lot of fat in the meat, obviously it is high in fat and should be avoided. Some cuts of beef and pork have less fat than others. These low fat cuts include beef round, flank, shoulder and rump, and pork loin.

Processed meat is usually very high in fat. Bacon, sausage, ham, hot dogs, and lunch meats contain enormous amounts of fat and definitely should be avoided. Processing the meat adds to the fat content.

Getting the fat out of your diet is an essential element of the Wellness Way to Weight Loss. As you begin to read labels and evaluate foods, you will see just how much fat you can eliminate from your diet. This fat elimination will help you to lose weight and will diminish your chances of becoming ill with a disease associated with the consumption of large amounts of fat.

TIPS FOR GETTING THE FAT OUT

- Give the fat test: Ask yourself, "Does it get hard?" If so, avoid it.
- Choose lean cuts of meat (eye of round, shoulder, rump, chuck, sirloin tip, round, flank, or tenderloin).
- Trim all of the visible fat off of the meat.
- Avoid marbleized meat.
- Choose poultry and fish; remove the skin.
- Use ground turkey instead of ground beef.
- Choose lean fish (cod, snapper, grouper, halibut, and shark).
- Use water-packed, not oil-packed, tuna

- Use only fat-reduced luncheon meats labeled "95 to 97 percent fat-free."
- Use nonfat and low fat milk and yogurt, fat-reduced cheeses, or cheeses made from part-skim milk.
- Avoid "hard" or aged cheeses.
- Plan dessert with frozen yogurt, ice milk, or sherbet instead of ice cream.
- Eat plain vegetables without butter and cream sauces.
- Use reduced-calorie mayonnaise, salad dressings, and spreads as condiments.
- Bake or broil foods to help reduce fat instead of frying, which tends to add fat.
- Grill foods; this reduces fat content as some of the fat drips away.

HOW COMMON FOODS COMPARE IN FAT CONTENT

Comparative Amount of Fat Content (in portions of 3½ ounces)

Highest fat	Liver
	Egg yolks (2 large)
	Hard cheese
	Red meat
	Poultry and shellfish
Lowest fat	White fish

HOW SALAD DRESSINGS COMPARE IN FAT CONTENT

Comparative Amount of Fat Content

Highest fat	Mayonnaise Blue cheese Thousand Island Miracle Whip Light Miracle Whip Ranch with mayonnaise	Lowest fat	French Ranch with yogurt Low calorie dressing (fat free) Lemon juice and vinegar

HOW CHEESES COMPARE IN FAT CONTENT

Saturated Fat in Different Types of Cheeses

Lowest saturated fat	Low fat cottage cheese Tofu (a cheeselike soybean preparation)
Low to medium	Ricotta Reduced-calorie cheese spread
Medium	Imitation mozzarella
Medium to high	Skim American Light cream cheese Part-skim mozzarella
High	Cheddar Monterey Jack Swiss Roquefort Canned cheese foods American Cream cheese Brie Cheese spreads

10

Fats and Disease

Just being overweight puts you at a greater risk of dying prematurely. Studies have shown that if you are 20 percent overweight, you have a 20 percent greater chance of dying at an earlier age than if you were at your optimal body weight. The same studies have demonstrated that if you are 40 percent or more overweight, then your chances of dying earlier increase by 50 percent. These are very alarming statistics.

Diets that contribute to obesity are diets typically high in fat. Being overweight not only contributes to disease and death but the fat content of your diet, by itself, can increase your risks of developing certain diseases as well. High fat diets have been associated with cancer, heart disease, stroke, and diabetes.

FATS AND CANCER

One of the most ominous fat-associated types of disease is cancer. "Cancer" is a word which scares everyone. Many times after making the unfortunate diagnosis of cancer, I will spend time talking with a patient and his or her family analyzing the type of diet the patient had been following. Time and again patients and their families have been consuming foods that were very high in fat for years, not realizing the possible damage they were doing to their bodies. Your chance of developing cancer could be markedly decreased by cutting down on the fat you eat.

The types of cancer that fat increases your risk for contracting include cancer of the colon (large bowel), cancer of the rectum, cancer of the breast, cancer of the uterus, and cancer of the prostate. Cancer of the colon and cancer of the breast are the leading forms of cancer in the United States.

There have been numerous studies comparing the rates of colon and breast cancer in populations that consume a low fat diet to cancer rates in Americans, who consume a typically high fat diet. All studies show a markedly decreased rate of colon and breast cancer in those populations which consume a low fat diet. Research suggests that there is a fivefold increase in breast cancer in those countries whose general population eats a high fat diet.

HOW HIGH FAT DIETS AFFECT YOUR RATE OF DEVELOPING CANCER

Foodstuffs high in fat move along your bowel at a slower rate then food which has less fat and more fiber in it. Because the fat-laden stool moves so slowly through the bowel, the stool sits for a longer period of time in your bowel. This exposes the bowel wall to possible cancer-causing agents in the food you have eaten. The slower the stool moves through, the longer the bowel wall is exposed to these harmful agents. This long exposure to cancer-causing chemicals is one theory explaining why high fat diets are associated with increased rates of cancer of the large bowel, and why people with chronic constipation also have higher rates of colon cancer.

The mechanism by which fats cause an increased rate of breast, bladder, and uterine cancer isn't as well known as cancer of the bowel. However, it doesn't really matter whether or not we understand the mechanism. What matters is our knowledge that high fat diets do put us at risk, and this risk can be avoided if we follow a low fat Wellness diet.

Although the mechanism is unknown, obesity alone is a risk factor for cancer of all types. This is especially true for cancer of the breast. The leaner you are (the closer to your ideal weight), the less chance you have of developing breast cancer.

FATS AND HEART DISEASE

The more saturated fat you eat, the higher the cholesterol level in your blood. Doctors are now absolutely certain that high blood cholesterol increases your risk for heart disease. Evidence also suggests that high blood cholesterol increases your chances of having a stroke. The mechanism for these increased risks is the build up of cholesterol plaques in the lining of your arteries. As the plaque build-up becomes larger, it interferes with the flow of blood to vital organs. One of these vital organs is the heart. Lack of blood flow to the heart leads to heart attacks. Another vital organ is the brain. Lack of blood flow to the brain can lead to a stroke.

FATS AND DIABETES

A diet high in fat also interferes with the body's regulation of blood sugar. Therefore, a diabetic who consumes a high fat diet will have a more difficult time with blood sugar control. The fat in the bloodstream blocks the receptors that the insulin binds to. The insulin has to bind to insulin receptors to keep the blood sugar in the normal range. When these receptors are blocked by fat, the insulin can't control blood sugar and the diabetic's blood sugar can get dangerously high.

The longer the diabetic's blood sugar is high, the more damage the diabetes does to the body. High blood sugar causes weakening of the arteries and veins, which leads to aneurysms. High blood sugar also causes atherosclerosis—blockage of the arteries. This weakening and blockage are why diabetics have a higher rate of strokes and heart attacks. High blood sugar also damages the eyes and kidneys.

WHAT TO DO ABOUT IT?

If you eat a diet high in saturated fats, the cholesterol in your blood is probably elevated and, therefore, so is your chance of having a heart attack or stroke. The goal, then, is to lower your blood cholesterol by lowering your intake of fat, especially saturated fats. What I highly recommend to my patients is a ban on the intake of saturated fats. As was discussed in Chapter 9, saturated fats include animal fats, butter fat, and tropical oils such as coconut and palm oil. This elimination, by itself, often drops their blood cholesterol level by about 35 percent. And with this drop comes a corresponding drop in the risk of heart attacks and stroke.

Heart disease is the number one killer of adults in the United States. Heart disease is associated with a diet high in fat. If the entire country went on a Wellness diet, the entire country would very likely improve its health.

11

Protein

The Meat-Eater's Mentality

Proteins are known as the building blocks of the body. Because they are building blocks, proteins are found in those areas of the body that "hold us together," such as our fingernails, hair, skin, muscles, and blood vessels.

Although proteins are necessary to a Wellness diet, there are many misconceptions about and just how much protein is required for good nutrition. The Wellness Way to Weight Loss includes consuming a diet made up of only 20 percent protein. This is a lot less than what most of us think is the "right" amount of protein for good nutrition.

Many athletes are taught that they should consume a lot of protein to build up their muscles. This is simply not true. Athletes, like anyone else, need only 20 percent of their diet to contain protein.

Americans eat more protein than almost any other nation. The typical American meal is "steak and potatoes." The potatoes are great but the steak is questionable. Most of us eat almost two times as much protein as we need on a daily basis.

PROTEIN AND YOUR METABOLISM

One of the main functions of protein is to aid metabolism. This means that proteins help the body in its daily energy production and utilization. Proteins also help regulate the body's water content and assist it in fighting off illness. Proteins fight off illness by helping the body build "fighter cells," which can attack foreign viruses such as the cold virus. In addition, proteins aid in the transport of oxygen through the blood and in hormonal regulation. Proteins make up a molecule called a globulin, which oxygen attaches itself to, and which is then delivered to other parts of the body. Proteins are part of the complex makeup of many of our hormones such as estrogen and testosterone.

However, too much protein can overload the body's filtering system. If we consume too much protein, this extra protein will be carried around in the bloodstream. The kidneys act as a filter for our blood. Too much protein "overloads" the filter and it becomes backed up. Individuals with kidney problems must adhere to low protein diets because their kidneys are very poor filters and protein rapidly "clogs" them up. Protein excess can also cause an increase in the body's uric acid level. Uric acid is a waste product and too much of it can lead to gout.

Too much protein can increase loss of calcium from bones and hasten the process of developing osteoporosis (weakening of the bones). This is especially true for women.

Some Problems with Proteins

Most of us were taught to eat meat and potatoes. We were taught that we needed protein to be healthy. The protein we were programmed to eat was usually high fat animal meat like rib-eye steak and pork chops. Other meats we grew up on were hamburgers and hot dogs—more high fat meats. These forms of protein are accompanied by a high level of fat and, therefore, increase your chances of developing the diseases associated with high fat intake, including heart attacks, strokes, and certain cancers. High fat also worsens diabetes and bowel diseases.

Not only do some meats contain large quantities of fat but other favorite proteins carry this extra fat as well. These high fat proteins include cheeses, eggs, and peanut butter.

PROTEIN AND YOUR WEIGHT

You probably eat too much protein. Too much protein, like too much of almost anything food-related, contains too many calories that could make you fat. Furthermore, a lot of the protein you eat probably contains excess fat.

But, protein eaten in the right amounts can aid in weight loss. One gram of fat contains 9 calories, while 1 gram of protein contains only 4 calories. This applies only to lean protein foods such as low fat cottage cheese and fish. It does not apply to high fat protein foods such as hamburger. Because of this difference in caloric value, if your diet contains the correct amount of protein it will contain less fat and, therefore, less of a concentrated source of calories. The end result is that you will lose weight.

PROTEIN AND THE WELLNESS WAY TO WEIGHT LOSS DIET

The Wellness Way to Weight Loss diet contains only 20 percent protein. For almost everyone this will be a great reduction in the amount of protein you eat. A small piece of meat (about a 3-ounce serving) contains almost one-half the total daily requirement of protein. In many of your diets the evening meal consists of much more protein than a small piece of meat.

Protein is an essential building block of the body. Thus, the Wellness Way to Weight Loss diet contains the essential amount of protein that is required by the body—no more and no less. This ensures Wellness on your way to weight loss.

Protein Alternatives to Red Meat

When you think of protein you probably think automatically in terms of meat—red meat. But there are other sources of protein, many of which do not contain as much fat. Fish is an excellent source of protein and one that is low in fat, cholesterol, and calories. Some vegetables, such as soybeans and kidney beans, are also high in protein content. Eating these types of proteins will allow you to get all the protein you need in a safe form. By including them in your diet, you will lower your calorie intake, which will lead to weight loss. If, in addition, you consume these proteins as the 20 percent protein complement of your diet, you will avoid the high fat proteins which will help to protect you from the risks associated with such proteins.

In general, the most important thing to remember is to cut down on your protein consumption and to specifically exchange high fat animal meats for low fat protein. Exchange highly marbled meats (steaks and pork) for lean meat (fish and chicken). These are excellent sources of good protein, protein that is low in fat and cholesterol.

An often overlooked source of protein comes from vegetable sources. Vegetable proteins are also very low in fat. The richest source of vegetable proteins are legumes—dried peas and beans. Fresh green beans and peas are not good sources because they have to be dried in order to concentrate the protein. Kidney, soy, pinto, and black beans are very high in protein, as well as black-eyed peas. Vegetable proteins are not, however, as complete as animal proteins. In other words, they don't supply the "complete" essential amino acids the body needs to make the building blocks it relies on. Although soybeans most closely resemble animal proteins, you should have some protein from animal sources in your diet.

If you decide to eat mainly vegetable protein, remember that you must eat a mixture of vegetables in attempting to get the complete protein you need. (Part of this protein should be derived from soybeans and added to other protein: dried beans, lentils, and split peas.) A common soybean preparation is tofu, which can be found in your grocer's fresh food section. It is very close to meat in the protein it provides. Another complete protein is wheat germ, which, like tofu, can be substituted for meat. The important thing to remember is to cut down on your protein consumption in general and, in particular, concentrate on eating those types of proteins that are low in fat.

12

Exercise

Energizing Weight Loss

Exercise is the key to both weight loss and Wellness. Exercise helps to alter your Fat Stat. You now know that the only way to lose weight and keep it off is to change your Fat Stat. Exercise burns calories, converts flab to muscle, and improves cardiovascular fitness. As a result, you will feel better, look better, and have more energy.

HOW EXERCISE EATS UP CALORIES

Exercising burns up calories. Not only do you burn calories while actually engaging in exercise, but if you exercise aerobically, you will burn extra calories for up to *two hours* after you stop. Exercise revs up your body's engine and keeps it that way for up to two hours after you finish exercising. This revving of your engine continues to burn calories faster than your body normally would, thus extending the benefits of the calorie-eating capacity of exercise. It takes two to three hours after exercise for your body to cool down. During this cooling-down period, extra calories are still being used as fuel. The longer you exercise and the more intense the "workout," the longer your body stays revved up and the longer it takes to cool down. So the formula for eating up calories that could turn to fat becomes elementary: intensity of exercise × length of exercise = number of calories burned.

For example:

Jogging (6 mph) × 1 hour = 564 calories burned

or

Walking (3 mph) × ½ hour = 170 calories burned

The more intense the exercise, the more calories burned for any length of time. An example of low intensity exercise would be walking or slow swimming. Medium intensity exercise would include jogging 12-minute miles, while running 7-minute miles or bicycling at 20 miles per hour would be high intensity exercise. Page 99 provides a list of exercises and calories that each burns per hour.

EXERCISE AND THE FAT STAT

What we all want when we diet is a rapid decline of weight. In other words, we want to look down at the scale and see the pounds sliding off—the faster the better. Exercise speeds up weight loss. By its very nature, exercise burns up calories and helps you lose weight more quickly. Exercise also helps overcome the body's tendency to slow down while you are consuming fewer calories in an attempt to lose weight—the Fat Stat at work. Whenever you lower your calorie intake, your body attempts to keep your weight steady instead of allowing you to lose weight. Remember how your body tries to sabotage your attempt at weight loss. It will try to keep the status quo, even though the status quo may include extra pounds that you don't want. The only way to combat this sabotage is to exercise. Exercise combined with calorie reduction will promote weight loss.

When you diet without exercise, a lot of the weight you lose, especially the initial weight, is lean muscle tissue. Obviously, when you diet you want to lose fat, not muscle. Exercising helps protect your muscle while encouraging a loss of fat. Fat is burned in your muscles for energy. If you lose weight without exercising, and lose muscle instead of fat, then you will ultimately decrease your body's ability to burn up that ugly, unwanted fat in the future.

EXERCISE MAKES YOU FEEL GOOD

Besides all the healthy benefits of exercise, physical activity helps you feel good. Exercise has been shown to increase the body's level of endorphins. Endorphins are chemicals in the brain that give us a natural high. The more you exercise, the more endorphins are generated and the better you feel. Many of us have experienced what I call the "diet doldrums." This occurs when you get tired of "sticking" to your diet. Exercise, because it gives you a natural high, also makes you more resolute in your stick-to-it-ive-ness. You feel good about yourself, good about your diet, and it becomes easier to continue eating in the Wellness way.

WHAT IS THE BEST EXERCISE?

There is no best exercise. Different people enjoy different activities. Some people like to walk; others like to run, swim, or bike ride. I personally find running to be the most enjoyable exercise, but I also enjoy swimming and biking. So there is no right or wrong answer to the question of what is the best exercise.

However, the exercise or group of exercises you choose must include a movement in which you use your larger muscle groups over and over again and on a continuous basis. Running, jogging, swimming, rowing, biking, cross-country skiing, and other types of "aerobic" activities are good because you move a lot of muscles over and over in a continuous manner.

Exercises like weight lifting, tennis, racquetball, and basketball are good but they aren't continuous. They start and stop. Therefore, they aren't aerobic—they do not require that you continuously move your large muscle groups. You can still enjoy participating in these activities, of course, but don't choose them to be the exercise that you expect will influence your Fat Stat.

Your preference for a certain exercise will certainly play an important role in your choice of activity. But other factors may enter into your decision as well when you are considering an exercise to do on a regular basis. Cost, environmental conditions, the condition of your body, and psychological factors should each be considered before you make your decision.

Cost

Some exercises cost money. Take striding on a treadmill, for example. To purchase a treadmill for your own use requires a considerable investment of money. Similarly, if you use the treadmill at a health club, the club's membership fee may also be costly. So if you enjoy using the more exotic kinds of exercise equipment such as the treadmill, stairclimber, electronic rowing machines, or electronic stationary bicycles, be prepared to spend money. You may want to investigate a club through a trial membership before you join on a permanent basis, which would be more costly.

Even an exercise like swimming can involve a cost if you live in a climate which requires that you swim in an indoor pool. Unlike outdoor pools, rarely are indoor pools public—either you pay a fee for the pool's use or a membership fee to a club which has its own pool. Sometimes these membership fees can be high. Local YMCAs or YWCAs may be worth looking into as their fees are usually somewhat lower.

Environment

If you live in an extremely cold area, then you must consider the effect of the cold weather on your choice of an exercise. If you are a bicycle enthusiast you will have a difficult time cycling when the chill factor is below zero. In that instance, it would be wise to have a second exercise you can participate in during severe cold spells.

However, almost any exercise can be enjoyed in almost any environmental condition as long as you dress appropriately. In cold weather it is important to layer your clothing. Two to three layers of light to medium clothing are much warmer and offer more protection than a bulky jacket. Remember to wear a hat and scarf. Up to 30 percent of your body heat can be lost through your head—more if you have thin hair or are bald.

Very hot weather can also pose a problem for exercising. This is especially true in areas plagued by high humidity. High humidity interferes with the ability of your body's sweat to evaporate. The evaporation of sweat is an important mechanism for cooling your body off. With the humid air already full of water, there is no place for the water produced by your body to go. So the sweat stays on you and acts as an insulator which keeps the heat in instead of taking it away.

Heat stroke and heat exhaustion are more likely to occur in hot and humid areas. As your body gets revved up with exercise, your muscles become heated and your body produces sweat. If the sweat can't help cool you off and you continue to produce heat, then you can get into trouble. To control heat-related illness, try to avoid exercising in the hottest part of the day—between 11:00 A.M. and 1:00 P.M. Also, it is vital to drink plenty of water to replace all the sweat you lose. Drink water both before and after exercising. Wear light and loose clothing which allows as much evaporation as possible and reflects the bright sun's rays.

Some people who are quite comfortable exercising outdoors in the winter find that walking or running outdoors during the heat of the summer can be unbearable. These people often walk in shopping malls, on treadmills, or on indoor tracks to avoid the heat.

Another environmental concern is the location of your activity. If you are a woman you must consider the possible dangers of exercising alone, especially at night. This is even more important if you live in or near a high crime area, although unfortunately no area is completely safe. If you are concerned, try to exercise only during the daylight hours and in areas that are well populated.

Another safe way to exercise is with a group. Running with a dog offers some measure of protection, depending, of course, on the size of the dog. I often ran with a friend's big Boxer. It was amazing how crowds would part when they saw me approaching with that dog at the end of the leash. All they saw was a big dog (the Boxer, not me) running toward them. They didn't know the dog's only offense would be to lick them to death.

THE CONDITION OF YOUR BODY

In addition to the issues of cost and environment already mentioned, the condition of your body may also determine which exercises you can or cannot do. Obviously, if you are just starting an exercise program, your body will rebel. Your muscles will get slightly sore and you will tire easily because you are not used to the exertion. Some conditions of your body, aside from the early aches and pains which will go away, may actually forbid you from doing certain exercises. If you have bad knees (either from old injuries or arthritis), running may be impossible for you. Fast walking may then be an alternative if you like to exercise outdoors. If you have circulatory problems and/or arthritis which are so severe that even walking is too strenuous, then you may need to seek alternatives such as swimming or bicycling. Heat- or cold-sensitive people should pursue indoor activities on an indoor track, pool, or exercising machine.

I recently developed a pinched nerve in my back—in the middle of triathlon season when I was in great shape. It was very frustrating when I had to give up running, bicycling, and weight lifting because my body wouldn't cooperate. But I did give it up, and I modified my exercise program to include only swimming.

If you have any questions at all about whether or not your exercise program would be harmful to your body in any way, talk with your doctor. Also, if you are over 35 and are about to begin an exercise program, you should talk the program over with your doctor. If you have any physical condition or disease, it is absolutely essential that you discuss any exercise program with your doctor before you begin.

Psychological Factors

This is an often overlooked area when determining which exercise program would be a good one for you. If you absolutely cannot stand running, cannot stand even the *thought* of running, then running is not for you. Similarly, if you hate the thought of getting your hair wet with chlorinated water three times a week, then choose something other then swimming.

Choosing an exercise that you can do consistently is a very important decision. Since exercise is the key to weight loss and weight maintenance, at least choose an exercise that you have the potential to enjoy after you get in shape. Remember, all exercise is hard when you first get going, but after you get in minimal shape, then you will want to enjoy the great things you are doing for your body—like improving your aerobic capacity and your appearance. So choose carefully. Try different exercises for periods of time. You can do one exercise certain days of the week and a different exercise on the other days of the week. That way you don't get tired of one and continue to enjoy both of the exercises. Some people bike and swim during the summer and walk during the winter when biking and swimming are impossible. In short, have fun and enjoy exercising. Choose something you like to do.

HOW FAST, HOW LONG, AND HOW OFTEN TO EXERCISE?

How fast, how long, and how often to exercise are the most frequently asked questions after an exercise has been chosen. These are important questions because each has an effect on the alteration of your Fat Stat.

How Fast?

The key to changing your Fat Stat depends on how fast you get your heart rate going during exercise. Certainly anytime you exercise (unless it is twiddling your thumbs), you will burn extra calories. But if you exercise faster, you rev up your engine even more and will receive all the benefits that have already been discussed.

When you exercise you are building up your aerobic capacity, which is the ability of your heart and lungs to push blood through your body at a more efficient rate. To build up this capacity you must speed up your heart rate. Aerobic capacity changes after you have exercised at a certain rate for a specific length of time. When I talk about rate I am not talking about running a 7-minute versus a 10-minute mile. I am talking about exercising at such a pace that your heart rate will increase to a certain level that will eventually change your aerobic capacity.

How to Determine What Your Heart Rate Should Be

There is a simple method to determine what your heart rate range should be. The formula is as follows:

> Subtract your age in years from 220. Multiply this number by 85 percent for the upper level of your target heart range, and 70 percent for the lower level. For example, for a 33-year-old, the upper level of the target heart rate range would be determined by $220 - 33 = 187$; $187 \times .80 = 150$. The lower level is determined by $220 - 33 = 187$; $187 \times .70 = 131$.

So, when this 33-year-old is running or cycling, he or she must run or cycle hard enough to keep his or her heart rate in the range between 150 and 190. (The numbers are rounded off for convenience.) If the heart rate stays in this range, he or she will know that they are effectively exercising, improving their aerobic capacity and influencing their Fat Stat.

At first glance you might think that this is a high rate for your heart beat. But when you realize that this is well below the maximum heart rate and your physician has approved aerobic and strenuous exercise for you, then you can be assured that you are most likely improving your body, not damaging it.

You don't have to run really fast to keep your heart rate in the proper range. A slow to moderate jog is plenty. For Wellness, an individual need only stay in the target heart rate range.

There are two places to check your heart rate — in your wrist and in your neck. After you are exercising for a period of time, stop and quickly reach to either your wrist just below your thumb or your neck at the angle of your jaw and feel your pulse, using your index and middle fingers. Take your pulse for 15 seconds. Multiply this number by 4 and you have your heart rate. As soon as you have your heart rate calculated, begin exercising again so as not to lose the continuous effect of the exercise.

How Often?

How often should you exercise? To change your Fat Stat and improve your aerobic capacity, you must exercise at least three times a week. Many of us choose to exercise more frequently to change our Fat Stat more rapidly and therefore lose weight more rapidly. Some people even evercise up to 6 or 7 times a week. It takes more exercise to lose weight than to just stay in shape from an aerobic standpoint. Certainly exercising daily is much more effective for losing weight than exercising less frequently. Start with exercising three times a week. For a gradual weight loss this may be all you will need. You should notice weight loss after a month. If not, exercise 4 to 5 days a week and recheck your progress.

A word of caution is needed here. When you exercise you build up muscles. Muscles weigh more than fat, so you might actually *gain* weight initially as you are gaining muscle. This doesn't mean you aren't losing fat—you are. Often at the early stages of dieting and exercise, a more effective method of measuring weight loss is to use body measurements. Certain areas of your body, such as your waist, will be shrinking—even when the scale isn't making much of a change.

There is a myth that if you build up muscle and then quit exercising, the muscle will turn to fat. This is not true. What will happen is that the muscle will shrink and the fat cells that surround the muscle will fill up with fat as you gain weight. So you are gaining fat, not changing your muscle to fat.

The good news is that after you have reached your goal weight, you can experiment with less frequent intervals of activity. Some people can maintain their weight loss by exercising three days a week while others still must exercise on a daily basis.

How Long?

This question is still somewhat in debate. I recommend at least 30 minutes of continuous exercise. This 30 minutes does not include warm-up or cool-down. The 30 minutes means a full half-hour of jogging, swimming, biking, or whatever continual physical activity you choose. Of course, you should discuss this with your own physician first. Many physicians recommend just 20 minutes of continuous activity. However, I have discovered that much faster weight loss occurs after 30 minutes.

Unless you are already in shape, you should not start out

with a 30-minute workout. I recommend starting out at 15 minutes. If your chosen exercise is jogging, this initial 15 minutes can be a combination of walking and jogging. What is important is that you keep moving. Jog for a distance, then walk a distance. Slow down if you find you become short of breath. Walk until your breath returns, then jog again. There is no magic way to breathe—just try to breathe in a regular pattern. For example, breathe on every second or third step. Some people are more comfortable breathing through their mouth and nose at the same time. Others are comfortable breathing either through their mouth or nose alone. Do what is comfortable for you.

When you start exercising, it may be hard to get your heart rate up to your target range. Don't worry; the more you exercise, the better shape your body will be in and gradually your rate will pick up and arrive at the target range.

When you have exercised for the proper amount of time, gradually wind down before stopping—don't just suddenly stop. By gradually slowing down, your blood flow slows to normal and redistributes itself to the body. When you exercise your blood flows mostly to your large muscles. As you slow down, it redistributes to your abdomen and other areas. Stopping suddenly before this redistribution occurs can cause you to feel faint, and also has been associated with an increased risk of heart attacks.

EXERCISES

Walking

Walking is the exercise that I most frequently recommend because it can be done anywhere at any time. Walking outside can be done in almost any weather conditions except ice. Walking outside allows you to enjoy the scenery and just makes you feel glad to be alive, lose weight, and relish your body's improvements.

The way that you walk is important. When I talk about walking in a manner to change your Fat Stat, I am not talking about leisurely walking or ambling. I am talking about power walking—the method in which you lean your body slightly forward and walk with a big stride and swing your arms with each stride. This type of walking will raise your heart rate. Ambling about and talking to people you meet along the way will enhance your social skills but it will not do a thing for your Fat Stat.

Walking can be done with another person or with a group of people. Walkers, if they are the same height, usually walk at the same pace, and so a conversation can be held during a brisk walk. Walking is also good because it is easier on the joints than exercises like running or jogging. There is less jarring of the joints, which helps avoid possible knee and hip injuries.

Walking requires no special clothing, other than cool clothing in the summer and warm layers in the winter. It is important to wear reflective clothing if you are walking at night. A good pair of walking shoes is crucial, and I recommend that they have ample support for active wear. There are many varieties available on the market.

Walking can be done anywhere. Many cities maintain dirt paths in woody areas which are wonderful places to walk. Many shopping malls now sponsor walking programs and allow walkers into the enclosed mall areas in the early morning hours before shoppers arrive. Many of these malls play special music during walking hours and have distances marked off.

Start power walking continuously for 15 minutes, and gradually increase the time by about 5 minutes each week. You may want to follow a route religiously day after day, or you may want to have a variety of routes.

Jogging/Running

This is my chosen exercise. It takes less time and burns up more calories per minute then does walking. However, I have had my share of problems because of running, including two knee surgeries. I should add that although most runners have experienced some injury, few are forced to undergo surgery. I still love to run.

Running is similar to walking in a variety of ways. Like walking, running can be done virtually anywhere outside. However, running on uneven ground, such as on paths through the woods, may pose a problem in that injuries such as ankle sprains may occur. If you hit an uneven area on the ground, or run downhill too quickly, you can twist your ankle and suffer a sprain.

Clothing should be appropriate for the weather. Layered clothing, as I mentioned before, is much warmer, lighter, and less bulky than a coat; so I recommend layered clothing if running in cold conditions. When temperatures are warm, light and loose clothing should be worn. Also, as in walking, when jogging at night you should take care to wear reflective clothing.

A good pair of running shoes is essential. The shoes should provide both cushioning and support, and should be changed every year or every 500 miles. Carefully evaluate your shoes as they become worn. If they appear to be less supportive or cushiony, replace them. A bad pair of running shoes can lead to injuries such as shin splints (pain in the front of your shins) and knee or hip pain.

Unlike walking there is no really appropriate method of jogging. Some people amble along, others have a smooth gait, while some jog with such an incredibly angular and distorted gait that you can hardly imagine they are jogging. It doesn't matter as long as you move forward. Some people move along barely at a snail's pace while others glide along at 6-minute miles.

However, the important thing to remember is that you only need to move fast enough to reach your target heart rate. When you first start a jogging program, you will reach your target heart rate very quickly. As your body improves you will be jogging at a faster rate.

Biking

Many exercising people enjoy biking. Biking is an outdoor sport that allows you to just enjoy being outdoors, savoring the air and wind as it rushes by your face. Also because bikers cover so many miles, a lot of scenery can be appreciated along the way. A problem with biking though is that it depends heavily on weather conditions. It is difficult to bike against a 5-mile headwind. Also, biking during a rainstorm can feel like you are biking in a hail storm as the rain pelts your body. Because you are moving along at a fairly high rate of speed, biking in cold weather can set up a chill factor against your body that makes the weather feel even colder then it really is.

The type of bike you ride—10-speed, gearless, or mountain—doesn't matter. What matters is that you bike continuously, maintaining your target heart range. This may be easier to do with a 10-speed bicycle, however, especially if you live in a hilly area.

Clothes for bikers, as with any other exercise, must be appropriate for the weather. I suggest wearing biker's gloves, which help prevent your hands and fingers from going numb while biking. This happens when the palm of your hand is pressed against the handlebars and the nerve is compressed. A lot of bikers have special shoes which fit against the pedals, but these aren't really necessary if you are biking to change your Fat Stat and not biking competitively.

There is no special way to bike, but, remember, you need to bike fast enough to raise your heart rate to the target range. This means that you don't bike socially—get out there and pedal. It is difficult to bike at a continuous rate in the city: you have to stop for lights, traffic, and pedestrians. So every time you get going at a good clip and your heart rate approaches the target range, you have to stop and start all over again. Therefore, I recommend biking in the country, where all you really have to worry about are farm dogs and an occasional car. This recommendation works well for those who have access to wide open spaces. I realize that if you live in a city this will be a major obstacle, but even in cities there often are bicycle paths in parks with beautiful scenery.

In addition to wearing weather-appropriate clothing, I strongly recommend wearing a helmet. Helmets protect you from head trauma, which is the most frequent killer of cyclists. Biking accidents happen quickly and without warning. Combine that with high rates of speed and you can find yourself in a dangerous situation. Wear a helmet.

Swimming

Swimming is a wonderful exercise. Unlike running and walking it is easy on the joints. If you have had knee, hip, or ankle problems, swimming is probably the best exercise for you.

Swimming can be done year round if both an indoor and outdoor pool are available to you. The only requirements for swimming are that you know how to swim, have a swimsuit, and have a place to swim. As in any other exercise, you need to swim at a rate that will elevate your heart rate to the target range. This requires swimming laps in a pool. Start out by swimming as many laps as you are comfortable with. Gradually, as your ability and aerobic capacity improve, so will your lap numbers. Increase the number of laps until you swim for 30 minutes. Then continue to swim for 30 minutes each time you exercise.

There has been a lot of press in the past few years saying that swimming "makes you fat." This is because there has been some research demonstrating that swimmers often put on a layer of fat as opposed to runners who exercised with the same intensity and duration as the swimmers. The body responds to being cold by trying to protect itself, and one way it protects itself from cold is to insulate itself with a layer of fat. The research suggests that if you swim in heated pools, then your body won't have to lay down fat to keep warm. However, if you swim so that your heart rate reaches the target zone, you will be exercising your large muscle groups and changing your Fat Stat in the way that you desire. You will lose weight and you will lose inches.

Aerobics

High and low impact aerobics have become a popular way to exercise. Aerobic dancing is particularly fun since it becomes a group experience. Very often, members of the group psychologically support and encourage each other before and during a class. Moreover, a large group working out together surrounds each member with a feeling of both belonging and partaking with others in a vigorous routine. High and low impact aerobics are an excellent exercise method *if* the aerobic part lasts at least 20 minutes. Talk with the instructor and ask him or her how long the warm-up and cool-down periods are, as well as the length of the aerobic portion of the workout. Participate in those programs that contain at least a 30-minute aerobic section.

Exercise Machines

A great number of people who desire to exercise would rather exercise indoors rather than outdoors. Fortunately there are many different types of indoor equipment available for these people. Some of the most common types are bicycles, stair-climbing machines, and rowing machines. All of these help you exercise in a continuous manner so that you can reach your target heart range. Again, the advantage of indoor exercise is that it is weather independent. An easy, inexpensive indoor exercise can be accomplished by putting your outdoor bike on equipment that elevates the back wheel. That way you can pedal away indoors and work out all year long. Such equipment is available at most sporting goods stores.

Nonetheless, I have found the biggest problem with indoor exercise is boredom. Unlike walking, jogging, or outdoor biking, you can't watch the scenery go by when you exercise indoors. Try to overcome this problem by watching television or listening to the radio. Try concentrating on these other interests rather than on how long you have exercised and how much time you still have to go.

Calisthenics and Weight Lifting

Calisthenics and weight lifting don't aid in weight loss because they are not continuous aerobic exercise. However, they can be of great help in improving your appearance. Calisthenics and weight lifting can be used to shape your body by exercising specific problem areas. For example, sit-ups can help flatten the stomach and certain leg exercises can help trim the thighs and buttocks.

CALORIES BURNED PER EXERCISE

Below is a table which contains many different activities and the calories that each activity burns per hour. The actual number of calories you burn depends upon both the intensity of the activity and your body weight. More calories are burned with more vigorous exercise and higher body weights. So use this table just as a general guideline.

Activity	Calories burned per hour	Activity	Calories burned per hour
Ballroom dancing	330	Painting at an easel	120
Bed making	234	Preparing a meal	198
Bicycling (5½ mph)	210	Roller skating	350
Bowling	264	Scrubbing floors	216
Bricklaying	240	Sitting and eating	84
Carpentry	408	Sitting and knitting	90
Desk work	132	Sitting and reading	72
Driving a car	168	Sleeping	60
Farm work in a field	438	Standing	138
Gardening	220	Sweeping	102
Golf	300	Swimming (leisurely)	300
Handball or squash	612	Tennis	420
Horseback riding	480	Volleyball	350
Ironing	252	Walking (2.5 mph)	216
Jogging (6 mph)	564	Walking (3.0 mph)	340
Lawn mowing (hand mower)	462	Walking downstairs	312

Source: Exercise information from Princeton Pharmaceutical Products.

Exercise is an essential ingredient in the Wellness Way to Weight Loss diet. Aerobic exercise burns calories where you are active and for a period of time after you cease exercising. Exercise modifies the Fat Stat, enabling you to lose weight and keep it off.

13

The Diet

The Wellness Way to Weight Loss Diet

Finally, the chapter you have been waiting for—one that actually deals with weight loss. You now know the most important components of good nutrition: eat a lot of fiber and carbohydrates and cut down on fats, proteins, and sugars. You are finally ready to get down to the business of losing weight.

The way the Wellness diet works is very simple. More calories must go out than come in for weight loss to be accomplished. The average weight loss on this diet is a minimum of two pounds per week. To accomplish this all you need to do is follow the prescribed diet. Generally, you will lose weight more rapidly at first. This is good because seeing the scale go down is a great motivator to continue the diet. To lose weight even more rapidly, I suggest increasing your level of exercise in conjunction with your use of the Wellness diet.

CALORIES AREN'T THE ONLY THINGS THAT COUNT

It is not simply the number of calories you ingest that helps you lose weight. The types of food these calories come from is also a crucial factor to weight loss. Let me emphasize, again, the basic axiom: *fat makes you fat.* Fat produces weight gain much more easily because your body converts the fat you eat into body fat easier than any other food. One of the most important things to do on a weight loss diet is to severely limit your fat intake.

Remember, to convert the fat you eat into body fat, only 3 percent of the calories you consume are needed. To convert carbohydrates into body fat, 23 percent of the calories consumed are required to serve as fuel for the process itself. This means that if you eat 100 calories of carbohydrates, 23 calories will be used by the body to process the food and the remaining 77 calories will be available to be stored. But if you eat 100 calories of fat, only three calories will be used to process it and 97 calories will be left to be stored as fat. Therefore, concentrate on eating carbohydrates.

Remember, don't just count calories. Three small pretzels and three small potato chips are not equal, even though they each contain only 33 calories. Most of the calories in the potato chip come from fat and fat calories are more fattening. *So the most efficient way to lose weight is to cut down on high fat/high calorie foods (whole milk, butter, and the like) and eat high fiber/high carbohydrate foods.* This diet shows you how.

STARTING THE DIET

At the outset, you will be presented with a series of diet plans. Each diet contains approximately 50 percent carbohydrate, 30 percent fat, and 20 percent protein. Each diet is tailored to the American Diabetic Association's recommendations. The diet plan you choose depends on your needs. To lose weight you start on the 1000-calorie diet. To maintain weight you follow the diet plan corresponding to your height and weight (discussed in detail later).

Start with the 1000-calorie diet. No matter how much weight you want to lose, on 1000 calories a day you will lose weight. Now, on the 1000-calorie diet you won't lose weight as fast as on a lower calorie diet—but you won't lose the muscle in your body as you would on those very low calorie diets either. In any diet that is lower than 1000 calories, part of the weight you lose is muscle, not fat. In addition to the problem of muscle loss, on a lower than 1000-calorie diet, you will have the problem of rapid weight gain once you start eating more normally. Therefore, a 1000-calorie diet is an appropriate level to ensure safe weight reduction.

Remember: The key to losing weight *rapidly* is to exercise more in conjunction with the diet.

WHAT DO YOU DO AFTER YOU HAVE LOST WEIGHT?

Eventually, after you have lost the weight you wanted to, what do you do next? This is where many diets fail. They don't tell you what to do to maintain your weight, so you go right back to your old eating habits and consequently right back *up* to your old weight. Not so here. The first step is to determine how many calories you should consume every day to maintain, not gain, weight.

After you have reached your goal weight, determine what your daily caloric intake should be. Once that is determined, choose the diet that most closely corresponds to this requirement. Now you have Wellness guidelines to guide you for the rest of your life.

CALORIE REQUIREMENTS TO MAINTAIN (NOT LOSE) WEIGHT

Calorie requirements are based on body size, height, age, sex, and activity level. Consult the weight table below.

Desirable Weights[a]

Men					Women				
Height		Frame			Height		Frame		
ft	in	Small	Medium	Large	ft	in	Small	Medium	Large
5	2	128–134	131–141	138–150	4	10	102–111	109–121	118–131
5	3	130–136	133–143	140–153	4	11	103–113	111–123	120–134
5	4	132–138	135–145	142–156	5	0	104–115	113–126	122–137
5	5	134–140	137–148	144–160	5	1	106–118	115–129	125–172
5	6	136–142	139–151	146–164	5	2	108–121	118–132	128–143
5	7	138–145	142–154	149–168	5	3	111–124	121–135	131–147
5	8	140–148	145–157	152–172	5	4	114–127	124–138	134–151
5	9	142–151	148–160	155–176	5	5	117–130	127–141	137–155
5	10	144–154	151–163	158–180	5	6	120–133	130–144	140–159
5	11	146–157	154–166	161–184	5	7	123–136	133–147	143–163
6	0	149–160	157–170	164–188	5	8	126–139	136–150	146–167
6	1	151–164	160–174	168–192	5	9	129–142	139–153	149–170
6	2	155–168	164–178	172–197	5	10	132–145	142–156	152–173
6	3	158–172	167–182	176–202	5	11	135–148	145–159	155–176
6	4	162–176	171–187	181–207	6	0	138–151	148–162	158–179

[a]The weights given in this table are for adults between 25 and 59 years of age and include a 5-pound clothing allowance for men and a 3-pound allowance for women; the height measurements include a 1-inch allowance for shoes.

Source: 1979 Build Study. Society of Actuaries and Association of Life Insurance Medical Directors of America, 1980.

To determine your frame size, place a measuring tape around the smallest part of your wrist. This will give you your wrist circumference. Divide your height by your wrist circumference. This will give you your "*r* value" to place in the following table:

$$r = \frac{\text{Height (in centimeters)}}{\text{Wrist circumference (in centimeters)}}$$

	r value	Frame size
Males	10.4 or greater	Small
	9.6 to 10.4	Medium
	9.6 or less	Large
Females	11.0 or greater	Small
	10.1 to 11.0	Medium
	10.1 or less	Large

Use the frame size determined here to place yourself in the correct frame size found on the weight chart.
Source: P. Lindner and D. Lindner, *How to Assess Degrees of Fatness*. Available from Cambridge Scientific Industries, 101 Virginia Avenue, Cambridge, Maryland, 21613.

To determine your daily calorie intake to maintain but not gain weight, multiply your ideal weight by one of the following factors:

Age	Women	Men
Under 45	10	11
Over 45	9	10

Adjust caloric requirements for age by subtracting 10 calories for each year over 25 from your basal calorie requirement. For example:

47-year-old female/small frame/5′4″ tall
140 (lb) × 9 (calories per lb) = 1260 (calories)

47 (years) − 25 (years) = 22 (years)
22 (years) × 10 (calories per year) = 220 (calories)
1260 (calories) − 220 (calories) = 1040 (calories) necessary for weight maintenance

This is the number of calories you should eat every day. So look up the diet that corresponds to that number of calories and follow it. After a period of time you will know your diet so well that you won't constantly have to look up what you are allowed and not allowed to eat. The diet should become second nature to you.

Remember, though, if you are exercising a great deal and lose a lot of weight, but then you quit exercising and continue to eat the same number of calories, you *will* gain weight back. Think about it and it makes sense. If you exercise and change your Fat Stat and then stop exercising, your Fat Stat will slip back to its old weight and you will be caught again in the vicious cycle of a low Fat Stat which sabotages your ability to lose or maintain your ideal weight. Therefore, you must continue to exercise.

EXCHANGE LISTS

The reason for dividing food into six different groups is that foods vary in their carbohydrate, protein, fat, and calorie content. Each exchange list contains foods that are alike—each choice contains about the same amount of carbohydrate, protein, fat, and calories. Measurements are in grams.

Each exchange is the amount of food contained in a certain portion. In other words, one exchange of a starch contains 80 calories, 15 grams of carbohydrates, 3 grams of protein, and a

Exchange list	Carbohydrate	Protein	Fat	Calories
Starch/bread	15	3	trace	80
Meat				
Lean	—	7	3	55
Medium fat	—	7	5	75
High fat	—	7	8	100
Vegetable	5	2	—	25
Fruit	15	—	—	60
Milk				
Skim	12	8	trace	90
Low fat	12	8	5	120
Whole	12	8	8	150
Fat	—	—	5	45

trace of fat. Now to see what kind of food is in an exchange of starch look at the exchange list for starch. One exchange of starch can be a ½ cup of dry cereal or a ½ cup of pasta, an ear of corn, and so on.

Your diet is made up of exchanges, and the number and type of exchanges is determined by the particular calorie diet that you are following. To lose weight I recommend that you start on the 1000-calorie-a-day diet. So for breakfast you should eat 1 fruit exchange, 1 starch exchange, 1 meat exchange, 1 fat exchange, and one milk exchange. Think of exchanges as portions of food. Therefore, on a 1000-calorie diet, to determine what you can eat for breakfast look to the fruit exchange list and choose an exchange of fruit to eat. Let us say you choose a medium orange. Next choose a starch exchange from the list of starches and do the same thing for meat, milk, and fat exchange lists. Exchanges are certain amounts of a food type. The term *exchange* is used instead of portion because portion sizes vary with the type of food while exchanges do not. For example, one exchange of starch is equivalent to another exchange of starch, but the portions may be different. One exchange of ready-to-eat bran cereal is contained in ⅓ cup of cereal while one exchange for other ready-to-eat cereals is contained in ½ cup. Therefore, if I told you to eat a serving of cereal you might be confused as to what a serving is — a ½ cup or a ⅓ cup. But there is no confusion as to what an exchange is: it is 80 calories, 15 grams of carbohydrates, and so on.

FIBER SUPPLEMENTS

I recommend a fiber supplement with each meal. This supplement should be in the form of the powdered supplements available in all drug stores and most grocery stores. I recommend two teaspoons of supplement be added to each meal. This can be done by either sprinkling the powder in or on the food or by mixing it in juice or water and drinking it. Fiber is essential in a Wellness diet. Even though you are taking a supplement, you still need to increase your consumption of fiber-rich foods.

1000-CALORIE DIET

50% Carbohydrates *30% Fat* *20% Protein*

Exchanges	*Example*	*Quantity*
BREAKFAST		
1 fruit	Orange juice	½ cup
1 starch	Toast	1 slice
1 meat, med. fat	Egg	1
1 fat	Margarine	1 tsp
1 milk	Skim milk	1 cup
Fiber supplement		
LUNCH		
1 lean meat	Tuna	¼ cup
1 starch	Saltine crackers	6
1 vegetable	Tomatoes	½ cup
1 fruit	Apple	1 small
1 fat	Mayo-type dressing	2 tsp
Fiber supplement		
DINNER		
2 lean meat	Chicken, baked	2 oz
1 starch	Potatoes, mashed	½ cup
1 vegetable	Broccoli	½ cup
Vegetable(s) as desired	Lettuce, etc.	As desired
From the free food list	Low calorie dressing	1 tbsp

1 fruit	Banana	½ small
1 fat	Margarine	1 tbsp
½ milk	Skim milk	½ cup
Fiber supplement		

SNACK

½ starch	Graham cracker	1 square
½ milk	Skim milk	½ cup

This diet contains 17.5 total food exchanges. The total food exchanges include 3 fruit exchanges, 2 vegetable exchanges, 3.5 starch exchanges, 4 meat exchanges, 3 fat exchanges, and 2 milk exchanges. If you eat the exchanges as identified, you can be assured that you will be eating a Wellness diet with 50 percent carbohydrates, 30 percent fat, and 20 percent protein, and which contains 1000 calories.

1200-CALORIE DIET

50% Carbohydrates *30% Fat* *20% Protein*

Exchanges	*Example*	*Quantity*
BREAKFAST		
1 fruit	Orange juice	½ cup
2 starch	Toast	1 slice
	Shredded Wheat	½ cup
1 fat	Margarine	1 tsp
½ milk	Skim milk	½ cup
LUNCH		
2 meat, med. fat	Chicken, baked	2 oz
1 starch	Ry-Crisp crackers	4 (2 × 3½″)
1 vegetable	Tomatoes	½ cup
1 fruit	Orange	1 medium
1 fat	Almonds	6 whole (dry roasted)
½ milk	Skim milk	½ cup
Fiber supplement		
DINNER		
2 meat, med. fat	Lean ground beef patty	2 oz
1 starch	Hamburger bun	½ oz
1 vegetable	Beans	½ cup
1 fruit	Peach	1 medium
1 fat	Mayonnaise	1 tsp
½ milk	Skim milk	½ cup

SNACK

1 starch	Popcorn, unbuttered	3 cups
½ milk	Skim milk	½ cup

This diet contains 19 total food exchanges. The total food exchanges include 3 fruit exchanges, 2 vegetable exchanges, 5 starch exchanges, 4 meat exchanges, 3 fat exchanges, and 2 milk exchanges. If you eat the exchanges as identified, you can be assured that you will be eating a Wellness diet with 50 percent carbohydrates, 30 percent fat, and 20 percent protein, and which contains 1200 calories.

1500-CALORIE DIET

50% Carbohydrates *30% Fat* *20% Protein*

Exchanges	*Example*	*Quantity*
BREAKFAST		
1 fruit	Grapefruit half	1
2 starch	Whole wheat toast	2 slices
	Flaked bran cereal	½ cup
1 fat	Margarine	1 tsp
1 milk	Skim milk	1 cup
Fiber supplement		
LUNCH		
2 meat, med. fat	Roast turkey	3 oz
2 starch	Saltine crackers	8
2 vegetable	Carrot/celery sticks	3 each
1 fruit	Apple	1 medium
1 fat	Margarine	1 tsp
½ milk	Skim milk	½ cup
Fiber supplement		
DINNER		
2 meat, med. fat	Broiled halibut	2 oz
2 starch	Baked potato	1 medium
	French bread	1 slice
1 vegetable	Green beans	½ cup
1 fruit	Papaya	1 cup
1 fat	Peanuts	20 small
Fiber supplement		

SNACK

1 starch	Pretzels	¾ oz
½ milk	Skim milk	½ cup

This diet contains 22 total food exchanges. The total food exchanges include 3 fruit exchanges, 3 vegetable exchanges, 7 starch exchanges, 4 meat exchanges, 3 fat exchanges, and 2 milk exchanges. If you eat the exchanges as identified, you can be assured that you will be eating a Wellness diet with 50 percent carbohydrates, 30 percent fat, and 20 percent protein, and which contains 1500 calories.

1800-CALORIE DIET

50% Carbohydrates *30% Fat* *20% Protein*

Exchanges	*Example*	*Quantity*
BREAKFAST		
2 fruit	Orange juice	1 cup
3 starch	Whole wheat toast	2 slices
1 fat	Margarine	1 tsp
1 milk	Skim milk	1 cup
Fiber supplement		
LUNCH		
2 meat, med. fat	Tuna	½ cup
3 starch	Rye bread	3 slices
1 vegetable	Green beans	½ cup
1 fruit	Orange	1 medium
2 fat	Mayonnaise	1 tsp
1 milk	Skim milk	½ cup
Fiber supplement		
DINNER		
3 meat, med. fat	Roast beef	3 oz
2 starch	Potatoes	2 small
1 vegetable	Broccoli	½ cup
1 fruit	Strawberries	1½ cup
1 fat	Margarine	1 tsp
½ milk	Skim milk	½ cup
Fiber supplement		

SNACK		
1 starch	Graham crackers	3
½ milk	Skim milk	½ cup

This diet contains 27 total food exchanges. The total food exchanges include 4 fruit exchanges, 2 vegetable exchanges, 9 starch exchanges, 5 meat exchanges, 4 fat exchanges, and 3 milk exchanges. If you eat the exchanges as identified, you can be assured that you will be eating a Wellness diet with 50 percent carbohydrates, 30 percent fat, and 20 percent protein, and which contains 1800 calories.

2000-CALORIE DIET

50% CARBOHYDRATES 30% FAT 20% PROTEIN

Exchanges	*Example*	*Quantity*
BREAKFAST		
2 fruit	Orange juice	1 cup
3 starch	Grapenuts cereal	9 tbsp
1 fat	Bacon	1 strip
1 milk	Skim milk	1 cup
Fiber supplement		
LUNCH		
2 meat, med. fat	Corned beef	2 oz
3 starch	Bagel	1½
1 vegetable	Corn	⅓ cup
1 fruit	Apple	1 medium
2 fat	Margarine	1 tsp
½ milk	Skim milk	½ cup
Fiber supplement		
DINNER		
3 meat, med. fat	Lobster	¾ cup
2 starch	Wild rice	⅔ cup
1 vegetable	Beets	½ cup
2 fruit	Applesauce	1 cup
2 fat	Sunflower seeds	2 tbsp
Fiber supplement		
SNACK		
2 starch	Popcorn	6 cups

1 meat, med. fat	Sardines	2 medium
½ milk	Skim milk	½ cup

This diet contains 30 total food exchanges. The total food exchanges include 5 fruit exchanges, 2 vegetable exchanges, 10 starch exchanges, 6 meat exchanges, 5 fat exchanges, and 2 milk exchanges. If you eat the exchanges as identified, you can be assured that you will be eating a Wellness diet with 50 percent carbohydrates, 30 percent fat, and 20 percent protein, and which contains 2000 calories.

EXCHANGE LIST FOR MEAL PLANNING

Starch/Bread List

Each item in this list contains approximately 15 grams of carbohydrate, 3 grams of protein, a trace of fat, and 80 calories. Whole grain products average about 2 grams of fiber per serving and are in italic type. Those foods that contain 3 or more grams of fiber per serving are marked with an asterisk (*) and are in italic type.

CEREAL

1/3 cup	**Bran Cereals*, concentrated (e.g., All Bran)
1/2 cup	**Bran flakes*
1/2 cup	*Bulgur* (cooked)
1/2 cup	Cereal, cooked (oatmeal)
3/4 cup	Cereal, ready-to-eat, unsweetened
(3/4 oz)	(Wheaties, Wheat Chex)
2 1/2 tbsp	Cornmeal (dry)
3 tbsp	Grapenuts
1/2 cup	Grits (cooked)
1/2 cup	Pasta (cooked), spaghetti, noodles, macaroni
1 1/2 cup	*Puffed cereal* (unfrosted)
1/3 cup	Rice, brown rice, barley (cooked)
1/2 cup	*Shredded wheat*
3 tbsp	*Wheat germ*

DRIED BEANS/PEAS/LENTILS

1/3 cup	*Dried beans, peas* (cooked) (kidney or navy beans, blackeye or split peas)
1/3 cup	*Lentils* (cooked)
1/4 cup	*Baked beans* (no pork)

STARCHY VEGETABLES

½ cup	*Corn*
1 ear	*Corn on the cob*, 6″
½ cup	**Lima beans*
½ cup	*Mixed vegetables*
⅔ cup	*Parsnips*
½ cup	*Peas, green* (canned or frozen)
½ cup	*Plantain*
1 small (3 oz)	*Potato, white*
½ cup	*Potato, white* (mashed)
¾ cup	*Squash, winter* (acorn or butternut)
⅓ cup	*Yam or sweet potato*

BREAD

½ (1 oz)	Bagel
1 slice (1 oz)	Bread (white, French, Italian)
2 slices	Low calorie bread (40 calories per slice)
1 slice (1 oz)	Bread (whole wheat, rye, or pumpernickel)
1 slice (1 oz)	Bread, raisin (no icing)
2 (⅔ oz)	Bread sticks, crisp (4″ × ½″)
1 cup	Croutons, low fat
½	English muffin
½ (1 oz)	Frankfurter or hamburger bun
½	Pita bread, 6″ (whole wheat)
1 small (1 oz)	Plain roll
1	Tortilla, 6″ (corn or flour)
¼ cup	Bread crumbs
2½ tbsp	Flour, cornstarch, tapioca

CRACKERS/SNACKS

8	Animal crackers
3	*Graham crackers*, 2½″ square
¾	Matzo, 4″ × 6″

5 slices	Melba toast
24	Oyster crackers
3 cups	*Popcorn* (popped, no fat added)
¾ oz	Pretzels
4	*Ry-Crisp*, 2″ × 3½″
6	Saltine-type crackers
2–4 slices (3–4 oz)	Whole wheat crackers, no fat added (crisp breads, such as Finn, Kavli, Wasa)

STARCH FOODS PREPARED WITH FAT (count as 1 starch/bread serving plus 1 fat serving)

1	Biscuit, 2½″ across
½ cup	Chow mein noodles
1 piece	Cornbread, 2″ cube
6	Crackers, round butter and snack type
1 small	Muffin, plain (bran)
10 (1½ oz)	French fried potatoes, 2″ to 3½″ long
2	Pancake, 4″ across
¼ cup	Stuffing, bread (prepared)
2	Taco shells, 6″ (corn)
1	Waffle, 4½″ square
4–6 (1 oz)	Wheat crackers with fat added (Triscuits)

Milk List

Each serving of milk or milk products on this list contains about 12 grams of carbohydrate and 8 grams of protein. The calories vary with the fat content of the milk. The milk list is divided into three parts based on the amount of fat and calories and is measured in grams. One serving from the milk list (one milk exchange) includes:

	Carbohydrate	Protein	Fat	Calories
Lean	12	8	trace	90
Medium fat	12	8	5	120
High fat	12	8	8	150

SKIM OR NONFAT FORTIFIED MILK

1 cup	Skim or nonfat milk (0.5%)
1 cup	1% fat milk
⅓ cup	Dry nonfat milk (before adding liquid)
½ cup	Evaporated skim milk
1 cup	Buttermilk made from skim milk
6–8 oz	Plain nonfat yogurt (check the label)

LOW FAT FORTIFIED MILK

1 cup	2% fat milk
6–8 oz	Low fat yogurt (check the label for fat content)

WHOLE MILK

Foods in the whole milk group are high in fat. They should be limited as much as possible.

1 cup	Whole milk
½ cup	Evaporated whole milk

Meat List

Each serving (ounce) of meat or substitute on this list contains about 7 grams of protein. The amount of fat and calories in protein foods varies, so the list is divided into three parts—lean meat, medium fat meat, and high fat meat—and measured in grams. One ounce (one meat exchange) of each of these includes:

	Carbohydrate	Protein	Fat	Calories
Lean	0	7	3	55
Medium fat	0	7	5	75
High fat	0	7	8	100

Use of lean meats is encouraged as much as possible, with medium fat meats used less often, and high fat meats only occasionally because of their tendency to contribute to increased serum cholesterol levels.

Guidelines for Preparing Meat

1. Bake, roast, broil, grill, or boil these foods rather than fry them with added fat. Let the fat drip away from the meat when preparing it.
2. Use a nonstick pan spray or a nonstick pan to brown or fry these foods.
3. Trim off visible fat before and after cooking, and remove skin from chicken.
4. Do not add flour, bread crumbs, coating mixes, or fat to these foods when preparing them (unless it is counted).
5. Weigh meat after cooking and removing bone and fat. A 4-ounce serving of raw meat (5 or 6 ounces with bone) is about equal to 3 ounces of cooked meat. Some examples of meat portions are:

2 ounces meat =	1 small chicken leg or thigh
(2 meat exchanges)	½ cup cottage cheese or tuna
	1 medium pork chop
	1 small hamburger
3 ounces meat =	1 chicken breast
(3 meat exchanges)	1 unbreaded fish fillet
	Cooked meat about the size of a deck of cards (3 oz)

6. Restaurants usually serve prime cuts of meat which are high in fat and calories.

Lean Meat and Substitutes

One exchange contains 7 grams of protein, 3 grams of fat, and 55 calories.

1 oz	Beef—USDA Select or Choice grades of lean beef (round, sirloin, and flank steak; tenderloin; chipped beef)
1 oz	Pork—Lean pork, such as fresh ham, canned, cured, or boiled ham, Canadian bacon; tenderloin
1 oz	Veal—All cuts are lean except for veal cutlets (ground or cubed)
1 oz	Lamb—Arm chop, loin chop, leg
1 oz	Poultry (remove skin)—chicken, turkey, cornish hen
1 oz	Fish—Any fresh or frozen fish
2 oz	Crab, lobster, scallops, shrimp, clams
6 medium	Oysters
¼ cup	Tuna (canned in water)
1 oz	Herring (uncreamed or smoked)
2 medium	Sardines (canned and drained)
1 oz	Wild game—Venison, rabbit, squirrel, pheasant, duck, goose (without skin)
1 oz	95% fat-free luncheon meat
¼ cup	Egg substitute
1 oz	Diet cheese (less than 55 calories per ounce as noted on the label)
¼ cup	Cottage cheese (low fat preferred)

Medium Fat Meat and Substitutes

One exchange contains 7 grams of protein, 5 grams of fat, and 75 calories.

1 oz	Beef—Most beef products fall into this category. Examples include ground beef, roast (rib, chuck, rump), steak (cubed, Porterhouse, T-bone), meatloaf.
1 oz	Pork—Most pork products fall into this category. Examples are chops, loin, roast, Boston butt, cutlets.
1 oz	Lamb—Most lamb products fall into this category. Examples are chops, leg, roast.
1 oz	Veal—Cutlet (ground or cubed, unbreaded)
1 oz	Poultry—Chicken with skin, domestic duck or goose (well drained of fat); ground turkey
¼ cup	Fish—Tuna (canned in oil and drained)
¼ cup	Salmon (canned)
1 oz	Cheese—Skim milk or part-skim milk cheeses, such as
¼ cup	Ricotta
1 oz	Mozzarella
1 oz	Diet cheese (60–80 calories per ounce)
4 oz	Tofu
1 oz	90% fat-free luncheon meat
1 oz	Variety meats—Liver, heart, kidney, brain, tongue, sweet breads (high in cholesterol)
1 medium	Egg—(high in cholesterol; limit to 3 per week)

High Fat Meat and Substitutes

These foods are high in saturated fat, cholesterol, and calories, and should be used only three times per week. Each ounce of high fat meat contains about 7 grams of protein, 8 grams of fat, and 100 calories. Omit one fat serving for each ounce of high fat meat.

1 oz	Beef—Most USDA Prime cuts of beef; ribs, corned beef, beef sausage
1 oz	Pork—Sausage, spareribs, deviled ham, ground pork
1 oz	Lamb—Patties (ground lamb)
1 oz	Fish—Any fried fish product
1 oz	Cheese—All regular cheeses, such as American, Blue, Camembert, Colby, Limburger, Parmesan, Roquefort, Swiss, processed cheese
1 tbsp	Peanut butter (contains unsaturated fat)
1 oz	Luncheon meat (e.g., bologna, salami)
1 frank	Frankfurter, turkey or chicken (10 per lb)
1 frank	Frankfurter (count as one high fat meat plus one fat)

VEGETABLE LIST (LOW CALORIE)

Each vegetable serving on this list contains about 5 grams of carbohydrate, 2 grams of protein, and 25 calories. Vegetables contain 2 to 3 grams of dietary fiber. Unless otherwise noted, the serving size for vegetables (one vegetable exchange) is:

½ cup of cooked vegetables or vegetable juice
1 cup of raw vegetables (raw vegetables are more bulky for the same amount of calories as cooked vegetables)

Artichokes (½ medium)
Asparagus
Bamboo shoots
Beans (green, wax, Italian)
Bean sprouts
Beets
Broccoli
Brussels sprouts
Cabbage, cooked
Carrots
Cauliflower
Eggplant
Green peppers
Greens (collard, mustard, turnip)
Kohlrabi
Leeks
Mushrooms, cooked
Okra
Onions
Pea pods
Rutabaga
Sauerkraut
Spinach, cooked
Summer squash
Tomato
Tomato juice
Turnips
Vegetable juice (V-8 juice)
Water chestnuts
Zucchini, cooked

A small amount of the above vegetables may be used as a garnish or seasoning. Limit to 2 tablespoons. Do not count as an exchange.

Starch vegetables such as corn, peas, and potatoes are found on the Starch/Bread list.

Some vegetables are low enough in calories to be counted as free foods. They are found on the Free Foods List.

FRUIT LIST

Each item on this list contains about 15 grams of carbohydrate and 60 calories. Fresh, frozen, and dry fruits have about 2 grams of fiber per serving. Fruits that have 3 or more grams of fiber per serving are preceded by an asterisk (*). Fruit juices contain very little dietary fiber.

The carbohydrate and calorie content for a fruit serving is based on the usual serving of the most commonly eaten fruits. Use fresh fruits or frozen or canned fruits without sugar added. Whole fruit is more filling than fruit juice and may be a better choice for those who are trying to lose weight. Unless noted, the serving size for one fruit serving is:

½ cup of fresh fruit or fruit juice
¼ cup of dried fruit

Fresh, Frozen, Canned Fruit (Unsweetened)

1 small	Apple
½ cup	Applesauce
4 medium	Apricots (raw)
½ cup	Apricots (canned)
½	Banana (9″)
¾ cup	*Blackberries
¾ cup	*Blueberries
⅓	Cantaloupe (5″ across)
1 cup	Cantaloupe (cubes)
12 large	Cherries (raw)
½ cup	Fruit cocktail
½ medium	Grapefruit
¾ cup	Grapefruit sections
15 small	Grapes
⅛ medium	Honeydew
1 cup	Honeydew (cubes)
1 large	Kiwi
¾ cup	Mandarin oranges
½ small	Mango
1 small	*Nectarine

1 medium	Orange
½ cup	Orange sections
1 cup	Papaya
1 medium or ¾ cup	Peach (raw)
½ cup or 2 halves	Peaches (canned)
1 small or 1 large	Pear
½ cup or 2 halves	Pears (canned)
2 medium	Persimmons, native
¾ cup	Pineapple, raw chunks
⅓ cup	Pineapple, canned juice pack
2	Pineapple rings
2 medium	Plums
½	*Pomegranate
1 cup	*Raspberries (raw)
1¼ cup	*Strawberries (raw, whole)
2 small	Tangerines
1¼ cup	Watermelon (cubes)

Dried Fruit

4	*Apple rings
4	*Apricots
2½	Dates
1½	Figs
3 medium	*Prunes
2 tbsp	Raisins

Fruit Juice

½ cup	Apple juice or cider
⅓ cup	Cranberry juice cocktail
½ cup	Grapefruit

$\frac{1}{3}$ cup	Grape
$\frac{1}{2}$ cup	Orange
$\frac{1}{2}$ cup	Pineapple
$\frac{1}{3}$ cup	Prune

FAT LIST

Each serving on the fat list contains about 5 grams of fat and 45 calories. The foods on this list contain mostly fat, although some items may also contain a small amount of protein. All fats are high in calories and should be carefully measured. Everyone should modify fat intake by eating unsaturated rather than saturated fats.

Unsaturated Fats

$\frac{1}{8}$	Avocado (medium)
1 tsp	Margarine
1 tbsp	Margarine, diet
1 tsp	Mayonnaise
1 tbsp	Mayonnaise, reduced calorie
	Nuts and seeds:
6 whole	Almonds (dry roasted)
1 tbsp	Cashews (dry roasted)
2 whole	Pecans
10 large or 20 small	Peanuts
2 whole	Walnuts
1 tbsp	Other nuts
1 tbsp	Seeds, pine nuts, sunflower seeds (without shells)
2 tsp	Pumpkin seeds

1 tsp	Oil (corn, cottonseed, safflower, soy, sunflower, olive, peanut)
10 small or 5 large	Olives (green and black)
2 tsp	Salad dressing, mayonnaise type
1 tbsp	Salad dressing, mayonnaise type, reduced calorie
1 tbsp	Salad dressing (all varieties)
2 tbsp	Salad dressing, reduced calorie*

Saturated Fats

1 tsp	Butter
1 strip	*Bacon, crisp
½ ounce	Chitterlings
2 tbsp	Coconut, shredded
2 tbsp	Coffee whitener, liquid
4 tsp	Coffee whitener, powder
2 tbsp	Cream (light, coffee, table)
2 tbsp	Cream, sour
1 tbsp	Cream, heavy
1 tbsp	Cream cheese
1 tsp	Lard, bacon fat, shortening
1 tbsp	Meat gravy
¾-in cube	Salt pork

ALCOHOL

If you use alcohol, you must substitute it as an exchange.

Beer (12 oz) is equivalent to 1 bread exchange
2 fat exchanges

*Two tablespoons of low calorie salad dressing is a free food.

Light beer (12 oz) is equivalent to ½ fruit exchange
2 fat exchanges

Wine (4 oz) is equivalent to 2 fat exchanges

Liquor (gin, rum, scotch, whiskey) is equivalent to 3 fat exchanges

FREE FOODS

A free food is any food or drink that contains fewer than 20 calories per serving. You can eat as much as you want of those items that have no specific serving size. You may eat two or three servings per day of those items that have a specific serving size. Be sure to spread them out during the day.

DRINKS

- Bouillon, fat-free broth
- Carbonated drinks, sugar-free (diet pop)
- Club soda
- Cocoa powder, unsweetened (1 tablespoon)
- Coffee/tea
- Drink mixes, sugar-free

VEGETABLES, RAW (1 cup)

- Cabbage
- Celery
- Chinese cabbage*
- Cucumber
- Green onion
- Hot peppers
- Mushrooms
- Radishes
- Zucchini*

SWEET SUBSTITUTES

- Candy, hard, sugar-free
- Gelatin, sugar-free
- Gum, sugar-free
- Jam/jelly, sugar-free (2 tsp)
- Pancake syrup, sugar-free (1–2 tbsp)
- Sugar substitutes (saccharin, aspartame)
- Whipped topping (2 tbsp)

FRUIT

- Cranberries, unsweetened (½ cup)
- Rhubarb, unsweetened (½ cup)

*Three grams or more of fiber per serving.

Salad greens

- Endive
- Escarole
- Lettuce
- Romaine
- Spinach

Condiments

- Catsup (1 tbsp)
- Horseradish
- Mustard
- Pickles, dill, unsweetened
- Salad dressing, low-calorie (2 tbsp)
- Taco sauce (1 tbsp)
- Vinegar

SEASONINGS

Seasonings can be very helpful in making food taste better without adding a lot of calories.

- Celery seeds
- Chili powder
- Chili sauce
- Chives
- Curry
- Flavoring extracts (vanilla, almond, and the like)
- Garlic
- Garlic powder
- Herbs, such as basil dill, thyme, mint
- Hot pepper sauce
- Lemon/lime
- Lemon/lime juice (4 tbsp)
- Onion powder
- Parsley
- Pepper
- Pimento
- Salt*
- Spices (cinnamon, nutmeg, paprika)
- Steak sauce*
- Soy Sauce*
- Wine, used in cooking (¼ cup)
- Worcestershire sauce

*If you are on a salt restricted diet do not use table salt. Limit your use of other high salt food items such as steak sauce and soy sauce.

COMBINATION FOODS

This is a list of average values for some typical combination foods.

AMOUNT	FOOD	EXCHANGES
1 cup (8 oz)	Casseroles, homemade	2 starch, 2 meat, 1 fat
$\frac{1}{4}$	Cheese pizza (15 oz or 10″)	2 starch, 1 meat, 1 fat
1 cup (8 oz)	Chili with beans* (commercial)	2 starch, 2 meat, 3 fat
2 cups (16 oz)	Chow mein* (without rice or noodles)	1 starch, 2 meat, 2 vegetables
1 cup (8 oz)	Macaroni and cheese	2 starch, 1 meat, 2 fat
	Soup:	
1 cup (8 oz)	Bean*	1 starch, 1 meat, 1 vegetable
$10\frac{3}{4}$ oz can	Chunky, all varieties	2 starch, 2 meat, 1 vegetable
1 cup (8 oz)	Cream	1 starch, 1 fat
1 cup (8 oz)	Vegetable or broth	1 starch
1 cup (8 oz)	Spaghetti and meatballs (canned)	2 starch, 1 meat, 1 fat
$\frac{1}{2}$ cup	Sugar-free pudding (made with skim milk)	1 starch
If beans are used as a meat substitute:		
1 cup cooked	Dried beans*, peas*, lentils*	2 starch, 1 meat

*Three grams or more of fiber per serving.

FOODS FOR OCCASIONAL USE

AMOUNT	FOOD	EXCHANGES
$\frac{1}{12}$ cake (2 oz)	Angel food or sponge cake (no icing)	2 starch
3″ square	Cake, no icing	2 starch, 2 fat
2 small	Cookies ($1\frac{3}{4}$″ across)	1 starch, 1 fat
$\frac{1}{3}$ cup	Frozen yogurt	1 starch
3	Ginger snaps	1 starch
$\frac{1}{4}$ cup	Granola	1 starch, 1 fat
1 small	Granola bar	1 starch, 1 fat
$\frac{1}{2}$ cup	Ice cream, any flavor	1 starch, 2 fat
$\frac{1}{2}$ cup	Ice milk, any flavor	1 starch, 1 fat
$\frac{1}{4}$ cup	Sherbet, any flavor	1 starch
1 oz	Snack chips, all varieties	1 starch, 2 fat
6	Vanilla wafers	1 starch, 1 fat

FOODS TO AVOID

Sugar, honey, syrup, molasses	Jams, jellies, preserves
Candy	Condensed milk
Pie, cake, cookies, doughnuts	Alcohol
Regular soda pop	Sweet liqueurs, cordials

The exchange lists are the basis of a meal planning system designed by a committee of the American Diabetes Association. While designed primarily for people with diabetes and others who must follow special diets, the exchange lists are based on principles of good nutrition that apply to everyone. Copyright 1986 American Diabetes Association, Inc., American Dietetic Association.

14

Recipes for Wellness

On the next page begins a collection of recipes that are appropriate for a Wellness diet. Each recipe contains no more than 8 grams of fat. Remember, your goal is a diet that contains no more than 30 percent fat. By following the exchange program, you will be assured of this.

Each recipe is followed by a breakdown per serving of its fat, protein, and carbohydrate content. After this breakdown you will find the exchange information for each recipe. The fat, carbohydrate, and protein breakdown will help you learn which foods represent these different nutrient types. The exchange information will help you to include these recipes in your total daily exchanges.

As you will see, there are many recipes presented in this chapter. Variety is among the many wonderful things about the Wellness Way to Weight Loss diet. From these recipes you will be able to eat well at your daily meals, have parties that won't destroy your diet, and simply enjoy eating.

PRECAUTIONS WHEN MICROWAVING

Do not attempt to operate the oven with the door open since open-door operation can result in harmful exposure to microwave energy. Do not defeat or tamper with the safety interlocks.

Do not place any object between the oven front face and the door or allow soil or cleaner residue to accumulate on sealing surfaces.

Do not operate the oven if it is damaged. It is particularly important that the oven door close properly and that there is no damage to the door (bent), hinges and latches (broken or loosened), or door seals and sealing surfaces.

The oven should not be adjusted or repaired by anyone except properly qualified service personnel.

SOUPS

Cream of Broccoli and Cauliflower Soup

9 servings, ¾ cup each

1	package (10 oz) frozen chopped broccoli
1	package (10 oz) frozen cauliflower
1	cup shredded potato
1	cup water
2	tablespoons chopped onion
2	teaspoons low-sodium instant chicken bouillon granules
¼	teaspoon pepper
⅛	teaspoon ground nutmeg
3	cups skim milk

In 2-quart casserole, combine all ingredients, except milk. Cover. Microwave at High for 15 to 21 minutes, or until vegetables are tender, stirring 2 or 3 times. Let stand, covered, for 5 minutes. Process half the vegetables in food processor or blender bowl until pureed. Repeat with remaining vegetables. Return to casserole. Blend in milk. Microwave, uncovered, at High for 7 to 13 minutes, or until heated through, stirring once or twice.

Calories	59	Cholesterol	1.3 mg
Protein	4.6 grams	Sodium	56.3 mg
Carbohydrates	10 grams	Calcium	122.6 mg
Fat	—	Exchanges	2 vegetable

Tomato Rice Soup

10 servings, ½ cup each

1 can (14½ oz) no-salt stewed tomatoes
1 can (12 oz) no-salt tomato juice
1 cup hot water
1 cup cooked brown rice (recipe below)
¼ cup thinly sliced carrots
1 tablespoon frozen orange juice concentrate
1 teaspoon low-sodium instant chicken bouillon granules
⅛ teaspoon pepper
Dash ground cloves
Dash ground nutmeg
1 cup frozen peas

In 2-quart casserole, combine all ingredients, except peas. Stir. Cover. Microwave at High for 10 minutes. Add peas. Re-cover. Microwave at High for 5 to 10 minutes longer, or until carrots are tender. Let stand, covered, for 5 minutes.

Cooked Brown Rice

1¼ cups rice
2⅓ cups hot water

Combine ingredients in a 3-quart casserole. Cover. Microwave on High for 5 minutes, then at 50% (Medium) for 12 to 15 minutes or until liquid is absorbed and rice is tender. Let stand, covered, 5 minutes.

Calories	55	Cholesterol	—
Protein	1.9 grams	Sodium	30.5 mg
Carbohydrates	12 grams	Calcium	4.1 mg
Fat	.3 grams	Exchanges	1 bread

Hearty Minestrone

4 servings, 2 cups each

1	medium onion, thinly sliced
1	tablespoon olive oil
$\frac{1}{8}$	instant minced garlic
1	can (14$\frac{1}{2}$ oz) no-salt whole tomatoes, cut-up
1	package (10 oz) frozen mixed vegetables
1	cup cooked Great Northern beans (recipe below)
1	cup no-salt tomato juice
1	cup water
$\frac{1}{2}$	cup cooked brown rice (see Tomato Rice Soup)
1	medium zucchini sliced $\frac{1}{4}$" thick
1$\frac{1}{2}$	teaspoons sugar
1	teaspoon low-sodium instant beef bouillon granules
1	teaspoon Italian seasoning
$\frac{1}{8}$	teaspoon pepper
1	cup hot cooked whole wheat elbow macaroni
$\frac{1}{4}$	cup grated Parmesan cheese

Great Northern Beans

1	lb Great Northern beans
6	cups hot water
1	medium onion, chopped
1	bay leaf

Sort, rinse, and drain beans. Combine beans and remaining ingredients in 5-quart casserole. Cover. Microwave on High for

10 minutes, then at 50% (Medium) for 1½ to 2 hours, or until tender, stirring twice. Let stand, covered, 10 to 20 minutes.

Calories	316	Cholesterol	5 mg
Protein	15 grams	Sodium	189 mg
Carbohydrates	54 grams	Calcium	169 mg
Fat	7 grams	Exchanges	2 vegetable, 3 bread, 1 fat

APPETIZERS

Tangy Topper

16 servings, 1 tablespoon each

1 cup low fat cottage cheese
¼ cup low fat plain yogurt
½ teaspoon fresh lemon juice

In blender container, combine all ingredients. Blend until smooth. Chill thoroughly. Use in salad dressings or as a topping in place of sour cream.

Calories	12.6	Cholesterol	1 mg
Protein	2 grams	Sodium	72 mg
Carbohydrates	.6 grams	Calcium	15 mg
Fat	—	Exchanges	free

Lentil Pate

26 servings, 1 tablespoon each

2 tablespoons snipped fresh parsley
1 tablespoon minced onion
1 clove garlic, minced
3 tablespoons reduced-calorie margarine
½ teaspoon low-sodium instant chicken bouillon granules
1 can (16 oz) pinto beans, rinsed and drained
1 cup cooked lentils (recipe below)
¼ teaspoon pepper
1 tablespoon sherry

In small mixing bowl, combine parsley, onion, garlic, margarine, and bouillon. Cover. Microwave at High for 1 to 2 minutes, or until margarine melts. Pour into food processor bowl. Add remaining ingredients. Process until smooth. Spoon mixture into small crock. Cover and chill until firm. Serve as a spread with unsalted crackers.

Cooked Lentils

1 lb lentils
6 cups hot water
2 cloves garlic, halved
1 bay leaf

Sort, rinse, and drain lentils. Combine lentils and remaining ingredients in 5-quart casserole. Cover. Microwave on High for 10 minutes, and at 50% (Medium) for 30 minutes to 1 hour or until tender, stirring once. Let stand, covered, 5 to 10 minutes.

Calories	30	Cholesterol	—
Protein	1.4 grams	Sodium	34 mg
Carbohydrates	4 grams	Calcium	2 mg
Fat	2 grams	Exchanges	1 vegetable

Turkey-on-a-Stick

10 servings

- 1/4 cup sliced green onions
- 1/4 cup shredded carrot
- 1 clove garlic, minced
- 1 lb ground turkey
- 2 egg whites
- 1/3 cup rolled oats
- 2 tablespoons no-salt catsup
- 1/2 teaspoon chili powder
- 1/4 teaspoon dry mustard
- 1/4 teaspoon paprika
- 1/4 teaspoon liquid smoke
- 1/8 teaspoon cayenne
- 10 wooden skewers, 6-inch

Coating

- 1/4 cup cornflake crumbs
- 1/8 teaspoon paprika
- Dash cayenne

Tangy Mustard Sauce

- 1/4 cup Tangy Topper (see p. 144)
- 1 tablespoon prepared mustard
- 1 teaspoon snipped fresh parsley

Mix together onions, carrot and garlic in 1-quart casserole. Cover. Microwave at High for 1½ to 2½ minutes, or until tender crisp.

Combine remaining ingredients, except coating and Tangy Mustard Sauce, in medium mixing bowl. Mix well.

Divide turkey mixture into 10 equal portions, using ¼ cup for each. Shape into about 3-inch oval loaves. Insert wooden skewer into each loaf.

Blend all coating ingredients on wax paper. Roll each loaf in coating. Arrange on roasting rack, skewers toward center.

Microwave at High for 6 to 9 minutes, or until turkey is firm to touch and cooked through, rotating rack once.

Let turkey stand for 3 to 4 minutes. In small bowl, blend all Tangy Mustard Sauce ingredients. Serve turkey with sauce.

Calories	115	Cholesterol	41 mg
Protein	16 grams	Sodium	197 mg
Carbohydrates	4.6 grams	Calcium	24 mg
Fat	3 grams	Exchanges	2 low fat meat, 1 vegetable

Chunky Salsa Sauce

26 servings, 2 tablespoons each

1 cup chopped onion
1 clove garlic, minced
1 can (14½ oz) no-salt whole tomatoes, cut-up
1 can (8 oz) no-salt tomato sauce
1 can (4 oz) diced green chilies, rinsed and drained
1 teaspoon ground cumin
½ teaspoon dried oregano leaves
¼ teaspoon dried crushed red pepper

In 2-quart casserole, combine onion and garlic. Cover. Microwave at High for 2 to 4 minutes, or until onion is tender-crisp. Stir in remaining ingredients. Microwave, uncovered, at High for 8 to 11 minutes, or until hot and flavors are blended, stirring once or twice. Chill at least 4 hours before serving. Serve as a dip or sauce with fresh vegetables or tacos.

Calories	9	Cholesterol	—
Protein	—	Sodium	4 mg
Carbohydrates	2 grams	Calcium	2 mg
Fat	—	Exchanges	free

Mexican Bean Dip

26 servings, 1 tablespoon each

½ cup chopped onion

⅓ cup chopped green pepper

1 clove garlic, minced

½ teaspoon ground cumin

¼ teaspoon pepper

1 can (15 oz) garbanzo beans, rinsed and drained, or 1½ cups cooked garbanzo beans (see below)

2 tablespoons water

½ cup seeded and chopped fresh tomato

In 1-quart casserole, combine onion, green pepper, garlic, cumin, and pepper. Stir. Cover. Microwave at High for 2 to 4½ minutes, or until tender, stirring once. In food processor or blender bowl, process vegetable mixture, beans, and water until pureed. Return to casserole. Stir in tomato. Cover. Microwave at High for 2 to 3 minutes, or until hot, stirring once. Serve as a dip or spread.

TIP: When using cooked garbanzo beans, increase water to 3 tablespoons.

Cooked Garbanzo Beans

1 lb garbanzo beans

6 cups hot water

1 medium onion, chopped

1 bay leaf

Sort, rinse, and drain beans. Combine beans and remaining ingredients in 5-quart casserole. Cover. Microwave on High for 10 minutes, then at 50% (Medium) for 1¾ to 2¼ minutes or until tender, stirring twice. Let stand, covered, 10 to 20 minutes.

Calories	16.5	Cholesterol	—
Protein	1 gram	Sodium	55 mg
Carbohydrates	2.8 grams	Calcium	—
Fat	.2 grams	Exchanges	½ vegetable

Pita Pizza Snacks

4 servings

- 2 whole wheat pita breads, 4-inch
- ¼ cup prepared Basic Tomato Sauce (recipe below), divided
- ¼ cup shredded, low-moisture, part-skim mozzarella cheese, divided
- 2 tablespoons chopped green pepper, divided
- ¼ cup sliced mushrooms, divided

Split pita breads in half. Toast. Top each half with tomato sauce, cheese, green pepper, and mushrooms. Place on paper-towel-lined serving plate. Microwave at 70% (Medium High) for 1½ to 2 minutes, or until cheese melts, rotating plate after half the time.

Calories	85	Cholesterol	8 mg
Protein	6 grams	Sodium	146 mg
Carbohydrates	9 grams	Calcium	104 mg
Fat	3 grams	Exchanges	½ bread, ½ med. fat meat

Basic Tomato Sauce

2 cups sauce

- 1 can (14 oz) no-salt whole tomatoes
- 1 can (6 oz) no-salt tomato paste
- ¼ cup grated carrot
- 1 tablespoon finely chopped onion
- 1 clove garlic, minced
- 2 teaspoons olive oil

1 teaspoon packed brown sugar
½ teaspoon Italian seasoning

In 2-quart casserole, combine all ingredients, stirring to break apart tomatoes. Microwave, uncovered, at High, for 10 to 15 minutes, or until sauce boils and flavors are blended, stirring 2 or 3 times. Serve over hot cooked pasta or use in other recipes, if desired.

Calories	312	Cholesterol	—
Protein	7.7 grams	Sodium	98.5 mg
Carbohydrates	50 grams	Calcium	—
Fat	9 grams	Exchanges	1 vegetable, 3 bread, 2 fat

MAIN DISHES

POULTRY

Herb-Roasted Chicken

4 servings

½ teaspoon grated lemon peel

½ teaspoon dried oregano leaves

¼ teaspoon crushed sage

¼ teaspoon dried marjoram leaves

¼ teaspoon pepper, divided

¼ teaspoon instant minced garlic

2½ to 3 lb sole broiler-fryer chicken

1 small onion, sliced

½ teaspoon dried parsley flakes

Mix lemon peel, oregano, sage, marjoram, ⅛ teaspoon pepper, and garlic in small bowl.

Gently loosen and lift skin from breast and legs. Rub herb mixture under skin. Replace skin. Place onion and bay leaf in cavity of chicken.

Secure legs together with string. In small bowl, mix parsley and ⅛ teaspoon pepper. Rub onto chicken skin. Place chicken breast side up on roasting rack.

Microwave at High for 18 to 24 minutes, or until legs move freely and juices run clear, rotating rack twice. Let chicken stand, covered, for 10 minutes before carving.

Calories	244	Cholesterol	157 mg
Protein	42 grams	Sodium	146
Carbohydrates	1 gram	Calcium	—
Fat	7 grams	Exchanges	3 med. fat meat

One-Dish Hungarian Dinner

6 servings

2 cups chopped cabbage
1 cup chopped onion
1 medium green pepper, cut into ½-inch strips
½ cup sliced carrots, ½-inch thick
2 tablespoons water
1 teaspoon paprika
½ teaspoon low-sodium instant chicken bouillon granules
⅛ teaspoon caraway seed
⅛ teaspoon dried dill weed
1 can (16 oz) Great Northern beans, rinsed and drained
1 can (6 oz) no-salt tomato paste
2 tablespoons frozen apple juice concentrate
½ cup light beer
2½ to 3 lb broiler-fryer chicken, cut into 8 pieces, skin removed
Paprika
6 teaspoons Tangy Topper (see p. 144)

In 3-quart casserole, combine cabbage, onion, green pepper, carrots, water, paprika, bouillon, caraway, thyme, and dill. Cover. Microwave at High for 9 to 12 minutes, or until tender, stirring once. Stir in beans, tomato paste, apple juice, and beer. Arrange chicken on vegetable mixture. Cover. Reduce power to 70% (Medium High). Microwave for 25 to 29 minutes, or until chicken near bone is no longer pink, rearranging chicken after every 10 minutes. Let stand, covered, for 5 minutes. Sprinkle chicken with paprika before serving. Top each serving with 1 tablespoon Tangy Topper.

Calories	226	Cholesterol	57 mg
Protein	25 grams	Sodium	206 mg
Carbohydrates	27 grams	Calcium	49 mg
Fat	5 grams	Exchanges	3 low fat meat, 1½ bread

Moroccan Chicken Stew

4 servings

- 1 cup sliced carrots, ¼-inch thick
- 1 medium onion, cut into ½-inch pieces
- 1 cup (¼-inch cubes) rutabaga
- ½ teaspoon ground coriander
- ¼ teaspoon ground cinnamon
- ¼ teaspoon cayenne
- ¼ teaspoon caraway seed
- ⅛ teaspoon pepper
- 1 medium zucchini, cut into ⅛-inch slices
- 1 can (14½ oz) no-salt whole tomatoes
- 1 cup raisins
- ½ teaspoon salt*
- 1 package (12 oz) frozen cooked squash
- 2 whole bone-in chicken breasts (about 12 oz each) split in half, skin removed

In 3-quart casserole, combine carrots, onion, rutabaga, coriander, cinnamon, cayenne, caraway, and pepper. Cover. Microwave at High for 9 to 13 minutes, or until vegetables are tender, stirring twice. Stir in zucchini, tomatoes, raisins, and salt. Set aside.

Unwrap squash and place on plate. Microwave at High for 4 minutes, or until defrosted. Add to vegetable mixture. Arrange chicken breast halves on vegetable mixture. Cover. Microwave

*To reduce sodium omit salt.

at High for 20 to 25 minutes, or until chicken near bone is no longer pink, turning chicken over and rearranging after half the time. Serve chicken with vegetable mixture on couscous, if desired.

Calories	233	Cholesterol	68 mg
Protein	20 grams	Sodium	346 mg
Carbohydrates	25 grams	Calcium	58 mg
Fat	2 grams	Exchanges	2½ low fat meat, 1 bread, 1 vegetable

Chicken–Vegetable Stew

6 servings

1 package (10 oz) frozen baby lima beans
1 medium onion, thinly sliced
¼ cup thinly sliced celery
¼ cup chopped carrot
2 tablespoons snipped fresh parsley
2½ to 3 lb broiler-fryer chicken, cut into 8 pieces, skin removed
2 tablespoons plus 1 teaspoon cornstarch
½ teaspoon lemon-pepper seasoning
½ teaspoon poultry seasoning
¼ teaspoon dried rosemary leaves
1 can (10½ oz) ready-to-serve low-sodium chicken broth
2 teaspoons lemon juice

Unwrap beans and place on plate. Microwave at High for 2 to 3 minutes, or until defrosted. Set aside. In 3-quart casserole, combine onion, celery, carrot, and parsley. Cover. Microwave at High for 4 to 5 minutes, or until tender, stirring once. Add lima beans.

Arrange chicken over vegetables. In 2-cup measure, combine cornstarch, lemon-pepper, poultry seasoning, and rosemary. Blend in chicken broth and lemon juice. Pour over chicken. Cover. Microwave at 70% (Medium High) for 25 to 33 minutes, or until chicken near bone is no longer pink and juices run clear, rearranging chicken and stirring sauce every 10 minutes. Let stand, covered, for 5 minutes.

Calories	322	Cholesterol	84 mg
Protein	35 grams	Sodium	152 mg
Carbohydrates	34 grams	Calcium	64 mg
Fat	5 grams	Exchanges	3 low fat meat, 2 bread

Summer Chicken Salad

6 servings

3 cups water
1 cup bulgur or cracked wheat
1 boneless whole chicken breast (about 12 oz), skin removed
1 cup seeded chopped cucumber
¼ cup chopped red onion
1 tablespoon snipped fresh parsley
3 tablespoons reconstituted natural butter-flavored mix
2 tablespoons pine nuts
1 tablespoon olive oil
1 tablespoon white wine vinegar
½ teaspoon dried basil leaves
⅛ teaspoon garlic powder
1 medium tomato, seeded and chopped
¼ teaspoon salt*

Place water in 4-cup measure. Microwave at High for 5½ to 7 minutes, or until water boils. Place bulgur in medium mixing bowl. Add boiling water. Cover and let stand for 30 minutes. Drain and press out excess moisture. Set aside.

Place chicken breast on roasting rack. Cover with wax paper. Microwave at High for 4 to 5 minutes, or until chicken is no longer pink, turning chicken over after half the time. Set aside to cool.

In 1½-quart casserole, combine cucumber, onion, parsley,

*To reduce sodium omit salt.

butter-flavored mix, pine nuts, olive oil, vinegar, basil, and garlic powder. Mix well. Cover. Microwave at High for 3 to 4 minutes, or until cucumber is translucent, stirring after half the time. Cut chicken into ½-inch cubes. Add chicken, tomato, and salt to vegetable mixture. Mix well. Chill for at least 2 hours before serving salad.

Calories	178	Cholesterol	23 mg
Protein	11 grams	Sodium	74 mg
Carbohydrates	25 grams	Calcium	—
Fat	3.6 grams	Exchanges	2 low fat meat, 1½ bread

Garlic Chicken with Pasta

4 servings

- 7 oz uncooked linguine
- 1 boneless whole chicken breast (about 12 oz), skin removed, cut into $\frac{3}{4}$-inch cubes
- 2 cloves garlic, minced
- $\frac{1}{2}$ cup reconstituted natural butter-flavored mix
- 2 tablespoons snipped fresh parsley
- $\frac{1}{4}$ cup skim milk
- 1 tablespoon grated Parmesan cheese
- $\frac{1}{8}$ teaspoon paprika

Prepare linguine as directed on package. Rinse with warm water. Drain and place in large serving bowl. Set aside.

In 1-quart casserole, combine chicken and garlic. Cover. Microwave at High for 3 to 5 minutes, or until chicken is no longer pink, stirring every minute. Drain. Set aside.

In 2-cup measure, combine butter-flavored mix, parsley, and milk. Microwave at High for $1\frac{1}{2}$ minutes, or just until mixture boils. Pour over chicken. Mix well. Top linguine with chicken and sauce. Toss to coat. Combine Parmesan cheese and paprika. Sprinkle over linguine.

Calories	260	Cholesterol	35 mg
Protein	21 grams	Sodium	281 mg
Carbohydrates	39 grams	Calcium	60 mg
Fat	2 grams	Exchanges	2 low fat meat, 2 bread

Curried Chicken

6 servings

$2\frac{1}{2}$ to 3 lb broiler-fryer chicken, cut into 8 pieces, skin removed

- $1\frac{1}{2}$ cups buttermilk
- 2–3 teaspoons curry powder
- $\frac{1}{8}$ teaspoon pepper
- Dash ground cinnamon
- Dash ground cloves
- 1 medium onion, thinly sliced
- 2 cloves garlic, cut in half
- 1 cup julienne carrots ($1\frac{1}{2} \times \frac{1}{4}$-inch strips)
- 1 medium potato, cut into $\frac{1}{2}$-inch cubes
- 1 medium green pepper, cut into chunks
- 1 cup evaporated skimmed milk
- 2 tablespoons cornstarch

In 3-quart casserole, arrange chicken. In small bowl, blend buttermilk, curry, pepper, cinnamon, cloves, onion, and garlic. Pour over chicken, lifting pieces to coat. Cover. Marinate for 30 minutes. Add carrots, potato, and green pepper to chicken. Cover. Microwave at High for 20 to 30 minutes, or until vegetables are tender and chicken near bone is no longer pink, turning chicken over and rearranging after half the time. Remove meat from bones. Cut into bite-size pieces. Set aside. Add milk to vegetable mixture. Remove a small amount of liquid and blend it with cornstarch. Stir into vegetable mixture. Microwave at High for 5 to 9 minutes, or until sauce thickens and bubbles. Add chicken to sauce.

Calories	186	Cholesterol	60 mg
Protein	23 grams	Sodium	390 mg
Carbohydrates	15 grams	Calcium	213 mg
Fat	4 grams	Exchanges	2½ low fat meat, 1 bread

Oriental Chicken with Peanut Sauce

4 servings

1 boneless whole chicken breast (about 12 oz), skin removed, cut into ½-inch strips
¼ cup sliced green onions
3 tablespoons reduced-sodium soy sauce
2 tablespoons lemon juice
1 teaspoon honey
1 clove garlic, minced
½ teaspoon peeled, grated ginger root
¼ ground coriander
⅛ teaspoon dried crushed red pepper
⅛ teaspoon sesame oil
3 tablespoons unsalted dry-roasted peanuts
1 package (3¾ oz) cellophane noodles
8 oz fresh spinach, trimmed and torn, about 6 cups
¼ cup shredded carrot

Combine chicken and onions in 2-quart casserole. Cover. Set aside. In 2-cup measure, combine soy sauce, lemon juice, honey, garlic, ginger root, coriander, red pepper, and sesame oil. Set aside. Place peanuts in blender; chop until fine particles form. Set aside.

Prepare noodles as directed on package. Keep warm on platter. Microwave chicken and onions at High for 2 to 5 minutes, or until chicken is no longer pink, stirring once. Add spinach. Re-cover. Microwave at High for 2 to 2½ minutes longer, or until spinach wilts. Stir.

Drain cooking liquid into soy sauce mixture. Microwave at High for 2 minutes to blend flavors. Stir in peanuts. Top noodles with chicken and spinach mixture. Pour sauce over chicken and sprinkle with carrot.

Calories	146	Cholesterol	34 mg
Protein	18 grams	Sodium	237 mg
Carbohydrates	7 grams	Calcium	94 mg
Fat	5 grams	Exchanges	2 low fat meat, ½ bread

Spicy Chicken Tortillas

4 servings

Marinade

2 tablespoons reduced-sodium soy sauce
2 teaspoons white wine
2 teaspoons olive oil
1 clove garlic, minced
1 teaspoon sugar
¼ teaspoon ground cumin
⅛ teaspoon cayenne
1 boneless whole chicken breast (about 12 oz), skin removed

Topping

1 medium tomato, seeded and chopped
½ cup chopped green pepper
2 tablespoons sliced green onion
2 teaspoons red wine vinegar
⅛ teaspoon cayenne
4 flour tortillas, 8-inch
½ cup Tangy Topper (page 144)

In 1-quart casserole, combine all marinade ingredients. Mix well. Add chicken, turning to coat. Marinate for 30 minutes. In small mixing bowl, combine all topping ingredients. Set aside.

Place chicken breast on roasting rack. Microwave at High for 5 to 8½ minutes, or until chicken is no longer pink, turning chicken over after half the time. Cut into thin strips. Place tortillas between damp paper towels. Microwave at High for 30 seconds to 1 minute, or until warm. Spoon one-quarter of the chicken down center of each tortilla. Add tomato topping and Tangy Topper. Fold in one end of tortilla, then sides.

Calories	202	Cholesterol	36 mg
Protein	20 grams	Sodium	440 mg
Carbohydrates	20 grams	Calcium	65 mg
Fat	5 grams	Exchanges	2 low fat meat, 1 bread, 1 vegetable

Chicken Chili

6 servings, 1 cup each

½	cup chopped onion
½	cup chopped green pepper
1	clove garlic, minced
1	can (15½ oz) kidney beans, rinsed and drained
1	can (14½ oz) no-salt whole tomatoes
1	can (8 oz) no-salt tomato sauce
1	can (8 oz) no-salt whole kernel corn, drained
2	tablespoons red wine vinegar
2	tablespoons Worcestershire sauce
1	cup cut-up cooked chicken or turkey
1	tablespoon packed brown sugar
1	teaspoon chili powder
¼	teaspoon dry mustard
⅛	teaspoon pepper

In 2-quart casserole, combine onion, green pepper, and garlic. Cover. Microwave at High for 2 to 4 minutes, or until tender-crisp. Add remaining ingredients, stirring to break apart tomatoes. Cover. Reduce power to 70% (Medium High). Microwave for 25 to 30 minutes longer, or until flavors are blended and chili is hot, stirring twice.

Calories	187	Cholesterol	13 mg
Protein	14 grams	Sodium	75 mg
Carbohydrates	22 grams	Calcium	—
Fat	1 grams	Exchanges	2 low fat meat, 1½ bread

Barbecued Turkey Breast

8 servings

4½ to 5-lb. bone-in turkey breast

Marinade

- ½ cup reduced-calorie Russian dressing
- 2 tablespoons Worcestershire sauce
- 1 tablespoon lemon juice
- ½ teaspoon liquid smoke
- ⅛ teaspoon celery seed
- ⅛ teaspoon pepper

Remove gravy package from turkey breast and discard. Place turkey in large plastic food storage bag in baking dish. In 2-cup measure, combine all marinade ingredients. Pour over turkey breast. Secure bag. Marinate in refrigerator for 8 hours or overnight, turning bag occasionally.

Remove turkey breast from marinade, reserving marinade. Place turkey skin-side down on roasting rack. Estimate total cooking time into 4 parts. Microwave at High for first minutes. Reduce power to 50% (Medium). Microwave the remaining first one-fourth of time. Turn turkey on side. Brush with marinade. A microwave at 50% (Medium) for second one-fourth of time. Turn turkey on other side. Brush with marinade.

Microwave at 50% (Medium) for third one-fourth of time. Turn turkey skin-side up. Brush with marinade. Microwave the remaining one-fourth of time, or until internal temperature registers 170 degrees Fahrenheit. Let stand, tented with foil, for 10 to 20 minutes before carving.

Calories	200	Cholesterol	80 mg
Protein	31 grams	Sodium	273 mg
Carbohydrates	1 gram	Calcium	22 mg
Fat	8 grams	Exchanges	4 low fat meat

Turkey Wild Rice Paprikash

4 servings

2	cups cooked wild rice
2	tablespoons slivered almonds
1	medium onion, thinly sliced
2	tablespoons reconstituted natural butter-flavored mix
1/4	cup white wine
2	teaspoons paprika
1/8	teaspoon pepper
12	oz turkey cutlets
1/3	cup low fat plain yogurt
1/4	teaspoon salt*

Prepare wild rice as directed. Stir in almonds. Set aside, In 2-quart casserole, combine onion, butter-flavored mix, white wine, paprika, and pepper. Cover. Microwave at High for 4 to 6 minutes, or until onion is tender, stirring after half the time. Add turkey cutlets, turning to coat with onion mixture. Cover with wax paper. Reduce power to 70% (Medium High). Microwave for 5 to 6 minutes longer, or until turkey is no longer pink, turning over and rearranging after half the time.

Place wild rice on serving platter. Remove turkey from cooking liquid and arrange on rice. Stir yogurt and salt into cooking liquid. Spoon sauce over turkey. Reduce power to 50% (Medium). Microwave for 2 to 4 minutes, or until heated.

*To reduce sodium omit salt.

Calories	198	Cholesterol	19 mg
Protein	13 grams	Sodium	205 mg
Carbohydrates	25 grams	Calcium	59 mg
Fat	3 grams	Exchanges	2 low fat meat, 1½ bread

Fish and Seafood

Salmon and Mushroom Loaf

6 servings

$\frac{1}{2}$ cup sliced fresh mushrooms
$\frac{1}{2}$ cup chopped green pepper
$\frac{1}{4}$ cup chopped onion
1 can ($15\frac{1}{2}$ oz) salmon, drained and flaked
1 can ($10\frac{1}{2}$ oz) ready-to-serve low-sodium cream of mushroom soup, divided
$\frac{1}{2}$ cup rolled oats
2 tablespoons wheat germ
1 teaspoon prepared mustard
$\frac{1}{4}$ teaspoon dried basil leaves
$\frac{1}{4}$ teaspoon dried marjoram leaves
$\frac{1}{8}$ teaspoon pepper

Sauce

Reserved cream of mushroom soup
$\frac{1}{8}$ teaspoon dried basil leaves
Dash dried marjoram leaves
Dash pepper

In 1-quart casserole, combine mushrooms, green pepper, and onion. Cover. Microwave at High for 2 to 3 minutes, or until tender-crisp, stirring once. Let stand, covered, for 3 minutes. Add salmon, $\frac{1}{2}$-cup mushroom soup, rolled oats, wheat germ, egg whites, mustard, basil, marjoram, and pepper. Mix well. Spray

8 × 4-inch loaf dish with vegetable cooking spray. Spread salmon mixture into prepared dish. Cover with wax paper. Microwave at 50% (Medium) for 16 to 25 minutes, or until center is firm to the touch, rotating dish twice. Let stand, covered, for 5 minutes. Loosen edges and invert onto serving platter.

In small mixing bowl, blend all sauce ingredients. Microwave at High for 1⅝ to 2½ minutes, or until hot and bubbly, stirring once. Serve sauce over salmon loaf.

Calories	178	Cholesterol	25 mg
Protein	17 grams	Sodium	390 mg
Carbohydrates	9.6 grams	Calcium	266 mg
Fat	7 grams	Exchanges	2 low fat meat, ½ bread

Garlic-Herb Fillets

4 servings

1	tablespoon water
1	teaspoon grated orange peel
$\frac{1}{2}$	teaspoon dried rosemary leaves, crushed
$\frac{1}{4}$	teaspoon, dried thyme, leaved
1	clove garlic, minced
$\frac{1}{4}$	cup snipped fresh parsley
12	oz fish fillets, about $\frac{1}{2}$-inch thick, cut into 4 serving-size pieces

In small bowl, combine water, orange peel, rosemary, thyme, and garlic. Cover with plastic wrap. Microwave at High for 1 minute. Stir in parsley.

Arrange fillets in 9-inch square baking dish with thickest portions toward outside of dish. Top with parsley mixture. Cover with wax paper. Microwave at High for 5 to 7 minutes, or until fish flakes easily with fork, rotating dish once. Let stand, covered, for 3 minutes.

Calories	142	Cholesterol	47 mg
Protein	15 grams	Sodium	46 mg
Carbohydrates	—	Calcium	16 mg
Fat	8 grams	Exchanges	2 low fat meat, $\frac{1}{2}$ fat

Linguine and Seafood

4 servings

7 oz uncooked linguine
4 oz small shrimp, shelled and deveined*
4 oz scallops, rinsed and drained*
1½ cups sliced fresh mushrooms
⅓ cup sliced green onions
¼ cup snipped fresh parsley
1 clove garlic, minced
2 tablespoons reconstituted natural butter-flavored mix
Dash cayenne (optional)
3 tablespoons grated Parmesan cheese

Prepare linguine as directed on package. Rinse with warm water. Drain. Set aside. In 2-quart casserole, combine remaining ingredients, except Parmesan cheese. Mix well. Cover. Microwave at High for 4 to 7 minutes, or until seafood is opaque, stirring once.

Rinse linguine with hot water. Drain well. Add linguine and cheese to seafood mixture. Toss lightly to mix. Cover. Microwave at High for 1 to 2 minutes, or until hot.

Calories	268	Cholesterol	33 mg
Protein	19 grams	Sodium	228
Carbohydrates	42 grams	Calcium	100 mg
Fat	6 grams	Exchanges	2 low fat meat, 2 bread, 2 vegetable

*Cut shrimp and scallops into bite-size pieces, if necessary.

MEAT

Mandarin Beef

4 servings

Marinade

2 tablespoons reduced-sodium soy sauce
1 clove garlic, minced
½ teaspoon sugar
¼ to ½ teaspoon finely chopped dried hot red pepper
⅛ teaspoon ground ginger
¼ lb boneless beef sirloin steak, 1 inch thick, cut into ⅛-inch strips

Vegetables

1 can (8 oz) bamboo shoots, rinsed and drained, cut into julienne strips
1 medium green pepper, cut into ¼-inch strips
½ cup shredded carrot
⅓ cup diagonally sliced green onions, 1-inch slices

In small mixing bowl, combine all marinade ingredients. Mix well. Add beef, stirring to coat. Cover. Marinate at room temperature for 15 minutes.

In 2-quart casserole, combine remaining ingredients with beef and marinade. Cover with wax paper. Microwave at High for 5 to 8 minutes, or until beef is no longer pink and vegetables are tender-crisp.

Calories	129	Cholesterol	32 mg
Protein	16 grams	Sodium	297 mg
Carbohydrates	5 grams	Calcium	—
Fat	5 grams	Exchanges	2 low fat meat, 1 vegetable

Oriental Beef Patties

4 servings

Topping

- 1 cup shredded cabbage
- ½ cup shredded carrot
- ½ cup fresh bean sprouts
- 2 tablespoons finely chopped water chestnuts
- 2 teaspoons reduced-sodium soy sauce
- ⅛ teaspoon five-spice powder
- ⅛ teaspoon salt*

Patties

- ¾ lb ground round
- 2 tablespoons fine dry unseasoned bread crumbs
- 1 teaspoon reduced-sodium soy sauce
- 1 egg white

In 1-quart casserole, combine all topping ingredients. Mix well. Cover. Microwave at High for 3 to 4 minutes, or until tender-crisp, stirring once. Set aside.

In small mixing bowl, combine all patty ingredients. Mix well. Shape into 4 patties, about ½-inch thick. Arrange on roasting rack. Microwave at High for 2 to 2½ minutes. Turn patties over. Microwave for 2 to 3 minutes longer, or until medium done. Let stand, covered with wax paper, for 1 minute. Spoon topping over patties.

*To reduce sodium omit salt.

Calories	170	Cholesterol	58 mg
Protein	19 grams	Sodium	268 mg
Carbohydrates	6 grams	Calcium	28 mg
Fat	8 grams	Exchanges	2 med. fat meat, 1 vegetable

Ham and Potato Dinner

4 servings

4	medium baking potatoes
8	oz fresh mushrooms, thinly sliced
2	medium tomatoes, seeded and chopped
1	medium onion, cut in half lengthwise and thinly sliced
1/4	cup snipped fresh parsley
3	tablespoons no-salt tomato paste
1 1/2	teaspoons low-sodium instant chicken bouillon granules
5/8	teaspoon dried marjoram leaves
1/8	teaspoon pepper
6	oz low-fat boiled ham, chopped

Pierce potatoes with fork. Arrange in circular pattern on paper towel in oven. Microwave at High for 10 to 14 minutes, or until tender, turning potatoes over and rearranging after half the time. Wrap in foil. Set aside.

In 1½-quart casserole, combine remaining ingredients, except ham. Mix well. Cover. Microwave at High for 7 to 10 minutes, or until onion is tender, stirring once or twice. Add ham. Stir. Re-cover. Reduce power to 50% (Medium). Microwave for 2 minutes longer, or until heated through. Cut each potato in half lengthwise. Serve vegetables and ham over potatoes.

Calories	187	Cholesterol	35 mg
Protein	7 grams	Sodium	163 mg
Carbohydrates	35 grams	Calcium	21 mg
Fat	2 grams	Exchanges	1 low fat meat, 2 bread

VEGETABLES

HIGH-STARCH VEGETABLES

Simmered Beans and Artichokes

6 servings

3 cups water
1 cup bulgur or cracked wheat (optional)
1 package (9 oz) frozen artichoke hearts
½ cup coarsely chopped onion
½ cup coarsely chopped green pepper
1 clove garlic, minced
1 tablespoon olive oil
1 can (16 oz) Great Northern beans, rinsed and drained
1 can (14½ oz) no-salt stewed tomatoes
½ cup white wine
1 tablespoon packed brown sugar
¼ teaspoon salt*
¼ teaspoon dried oregano leaves
⅛ teaspoon dried marjoram leaves
1 medium white potato, cut in half lengthwise and sliced ¼-inch thick

Place water in 4-cup measure. Microwave at High for 5½ to 7½ minutes, or until water boils. Place bulgur in medium mixing bowl. Add boiling water. Cover and let stand for 30 minutes to soften. Drain and press out excess moisture. Set aside.

*To reduce sodium omit salt.

In 2-quart casserole, combine artichoke hearts, onion, green pepper, garlic, and olive oil. Cover. Microwave at High for 6 to 9 minutes, or until onion is tender-crisp, stirring once. Stir in remaining ingredients, except bulgur and potato. Re-cover. Microwave at High for 5 to 8 minutes, or until bubbly around edges. Stir in potato. Re-cover. Microwave at High for 15 to 25 minutes longer, or until potato is tender. Serve over bulgur, if desired.

Calories	281	Cholesterol	—
Protein	9 grams	Sodium	122 mg
Carbohydrates	53 grams	Calcium	35 mg
Fat	3 grams	Exchanges	2 vegetable, 3 bread, ½ fat

Herbed Summer Stew

4 servings, 2 cups each

1	can (16 oz) Great Northern beans, rinsed and drained
1	can (16 oz) pinto beans, rinsed and drained
2	cups sliced yellow squash, ¼-inch thick
1½	cups frozen cut green beans
1½	cups sliced fresh mushrooms
1	medium onion, thinly sliced
1½	cups cooked brown rice (page 141)
1	can (10½ oz) ready-to-serve low-sodium chicken broth
¼	cup white wine
2	teaspoons olive oil
2	teaspoons white wine vinegar
1	teaspoon dried basil leaves
½	teaspoon dried marjoram leaves

In 3-quart casserole, combine all ingredients. Mix well. Cover. Microwave at High for 15 to 20 minutes, or until hot and flavors are blended, stirring 2 or 3 times.

Calories	422	Cholesterol	4 mg
Protein	21 grams	Sodium	185 mg
Carbohydrates	74 grams	Calcium	102
Fat	6 grams	Exchanges	2 low fat meat, 4 bread

Slim Twice-Baked Potatoes

4 servings

2	medium baking potatoes
¼	cup dry curd cottage cheese
¼	cup buttermilk
2	teaspoons dry natural butter-flavored mix
1	teaspoon snipped fresh parsley
½	teaspoon freeze-dried chives
¼	teaspoon onion powder
	Dash pepper
2	teaspoons bacon-flavored soy bits, divided

Pierce potatoes with fork. Arrange on paper towel. Microwave at High for 6½ to 8 minutes, or until tender, turning potatoes over and rearranging after half the time. Wrap in foil. Let stand for 10 minutes.

Cut each potato in half lengthwise. Scoop out pulp, leaving ¼-inch shell. Place pulp in medium mixing bowl. Arrange shells on paper towel-lined plate. Set aside.

In food processor or blender bowl, combine cottage cheese and buttermilk. Process until smooth. In medium mixing bowl, combine potato pulp, cottage cheese mixture, butter-flavored mix, parsley, chives, onion powder, and pepper. Beat until smooth and fluffy. Spoon mixture into potato shells. Microwave at High for 3 to 4 minutes, or until heated through, rotating plate once. Sprinkle with bacon-flavored bits.

Calories	96	Cholesterol	1 mg
Protein	4 grams	Sodium	92 mg
Carbohydrates	19 grams	Calcium	—
Fat	1 grams	Exchanges	1 bread, 1 vegetable

Low-Starch Vegetables

French Green Beans and Pears

4 servings

- 2 tablespoons chopped pecans
- 1 tablespoon reduced-calorie margarine
- 1 package (10 oz) frozen French-style green beans
- $\frac{1}{4}$ teaspoon dried summer savory leaves
- 1 can ($8\frac{1}{2}$ oz) unsweetened pear slices, drained

In $1\frac{1}{2}$-quart casserole, combine pecans and margarine. Microwave at High for $1\frac{1}{2}$ to 2 minutes, or until margarine melts. Add beans and summer savory. Re-cover. Microwave at High for 4 minutes. Stir to break beans apart. Add pears. Re-cover. Microwave at High for 2 to 3 minutes longer, or until beans are tender.

Calories	83	Cholesterol	—
Protein	1 gram	Sodium	29 mg
Carbohydrates	12 grams	Calcium	—
Fat	6 grams	Exchanges	1 vegetable, $\frac{1}{2}$ fruit, 1 fat

Mediterranean Broccoli and Carrot

4 servings

1½ cups water
⅓ cup bulgur or cracked wheat
½ lb fresh broccoli, cut into flowerets, about 2 cups
½ cup chopped carrot
¼ cup sliced green onions
1 tablespoon reduced-calorie margarine
¼ teaspoon curry powder
1 tablespoon unsalted sunflower nuts

Place water in 2-cup measure. Microwave at High for 2 to 5 minutes, or until water boils. Place bulgur in small mixing bowl. Add boiling water. Cover and let stand for 30 minutes to soften. Drain and press out excess moisture. Set aside.

In 1½-quart casserole, combine all ingredients, except bulgur and sunflower nuts. Mix well. Cover. Microwave at High for 5 to 8 minutes, or until vegetables are tender, stirring twice. Stir in bulgur and sunflower nuts. Re-cover. Microwave at High for 2 minutes longer, or until heated through.

Calories	135	Cholesterol	—
Protein	4 grams	Sodium	42 mg
Carbohydrates	20 grams	Calcium	97 mg
Fat	5 grams	Exchanges	1 vegetable, 1 bread, 1 fat

Spiced Red Cabbage

4 servings

2 tablespoons apple juice
1 tablespoon packed brown sugar
2 teaspoons cider vinegar
¼ teaspoon salt*
⅛ teaspoon ground cinnamon
Dash ground cloves
4 cups shredded cabbage
½ cup chopped apple
¼ cup chopped onion
1 tablespoon reduced-calorie margarine

In 2-quart casserole, blend apple juice, sugar, vinegar, salt, cinnamon, and cloves. Add remaining ingredients. Mix well. Cover. Microwave at High for 8 to 12 minutes, or until tender-crisp, stirring twice. Let stand, covered, for 3 minutes.

Calories	91	Cholesterol	–
Protein	1 gram	Sodium	163 mg
Carbohydrates	13 grams	Calcium	–
Fat	4 grams	Exchanges	1 bread, ½ fat

*To reduce sodium omit salt.

Summer Vegetable Combo

6 servings

1	package (10 oz) frozen cut green beans
8	oz. crookneck squash, sliced ¼-inch thick
2	tablespoons water
2	tablespoons reduced-calorie margarine
½	teaspoon dried parsley flakes
¼	teaspoon onion powder
⅛	teaspoon dried oregano leaves
⅛	teaspoon garlic powder
	Dash pepper

In 1½-quart casserole, combine beans, squash, and water. Cover. Microwave at High for 7 to 11 minutes, or until vegetables are tender-crisp, stirring twice. Set vegetables aside.

In 1-cup measure, combine remaining ingredients. Mix well. Microwave at 70% (Medium High) for 20 to 30 seconds, or just until margarine melts. Drain vegetables. Pour margarine mixture over vegetables. Stir to coat.

Calories	57	Cholesterol	–
Protein	2 grams	Sodium	39 mg
Carbohydrates	7 grams	Calcium	43 mg
Fat	5 grams	Exchanges	1 vegetable, 1 fat

PASTA AND GRAINS

Hot Pasta Salad

4 servings

1 medium green pepper, cut into ¼-inch strips
½ medium red onion, cut in half lengthwise and thinly sliced
2 tablespoons reconstituted natural butter-flavored mix
2 teaspoons poppy seed
⅛ teaspoon salt*
¾ cup cooked spaghetti
1 medium tomato, cut into thin wedges

In 1-quart casserole, combine all ingredients, except spaghetti and tomato. Cover. Microwave at High for 3 to 5 minutes, or just until pepper and onion are tender, stirring once. Add remaining ingredients. Toss lightly. Re-cover. Microwave at High for 2 to 3 minutes longer, or until hot. Let stand, covered, for 1 minute.

Calories	65	Cholesterol	—
Protein	2 grams	Sodium	115 mg
Carbohydrates	14 grams	Calcium	—
Fat	—	Exchanges	1 bread

*To reduce sodium omit salt.

Barley Rice Pilaf

6 servings

- $\frac{1}{3}$ cup quick-cooking barley
- $\frac{1}{4}$ cup uncooked brown rice
- $1\frac{2}{3}$ cups hot water
- 1 cup sliced fresh mushrooms
- $\frac{1}{4}$ cup ($\frac{1}{4}$-inch cubes) carrot
- 2 tablespoons snipped fresh parsley
- 1 clove garlic, minced
- 1 teaspoon lemon juice
- $\frac{1}{2}$ teaspoon dried thyme leaves

In 2-quart casserole, combine all ingredients. Mix well. Cover. Microwave at High for 5 minutes. Reduce power to 50% (Medium). Microwave for 35 to 45 minutes longer, or until liquid is absorbed and rice is tender. Let stand, covered, for 5 minutes.

Calories	62	Cholesterol	—
Protein	1.6 grams	Sodium	7 mg
Carbohydrates	13.6 grams	Calcium	—
Fat	.3 grams	Exchanges	1 bread

DESSERTS

Cold Mandarin-Pineapple Souffle

6 servings

1 can (16 oz) mandarin oranges, drained (reserve 6 segments)

½ cup canned unsweetened crushed pineapple

½ teaspoon vanilla

1 envelope unflavored gelatin

½ cup water

2 egg whites, room temperature

2 tablespoons sugar

In food processor or blender bowl, process oranges, pineapple, and vanilla until pureed. Place ½-cup puree in small mixing bowl. Sprinkle gelatin over puree in bowl. Let stand for 2 minutes to soften. Reserve remaining puree.

Place water in 1-cup measure. Microwave at High for 45 seconds to 1¼ minutes, or until water boils. Add to gelatin mixture. Stir under gelatin dissolves. Stir in reserved puree. Chill until slightly thickened. To "quick-set," place in freezer for 15 to 20 minutes, stirring 2 or 3 times.

In medium mixing bowl, beat egg whites at high speed of electric mixer until foamy. Beat in sugar, 1 tablespoon at a time, until stiff peaks form. Fold fruit mixture into egg whites. Spoon into six individual dishes. Garnish with reserved orange segments. Chill for at least 2 hours, or until set. Refrigerate for no longer than 2 days.

Calories	65	Cholesterol	—
Protein	2 grams	Sodium	20 mg
Carbohydrates	15 grams	Calcium	—
Fat	—	Exchanges	1½ fruit

Raspberry Cheese Cooler

10 servings

3 oz Neufchatel cheese or low-calorie cream cheese

1 envelope (1.4 oz) whipped dessert topping mix, using skim milk

1½ cups water

1 package (6 oz) sugar-free raspberry gelatin

1 can (12 oz) sugar-free lemon-lime soda

2 cups frozen unsweetened raspberries

Place cheese in small bowl. Microwave at 50% (Medium) for 30 seconds to 1 minute, or until cheese softens. Stir until smooth. Set aside. In small mixing bowl, prepare dessert topping as directed on package, using skim milk. Beat in softened cheese. Set aside.

Place water in 2-cup measure. Microwave at High for 4 to 6 minutes, or until water boils. Place gelatin in large mixing bowl. Add boiling water. Stir until gelatin dissolves. Stir in soda. Blend ½-cup gelatin mixture into topping mixture. Set aside. Add raspberries to remaining gelatin mixture. Chill until slightly thickened. Pour into 9-inch round baking dish. Spread topping evenly over gelatin. Chill for about 3 hours, or until set. Cut into wedges.

Calories	70	Cholesterol	11 mg
Protein	3 grams	Sodium	25 mg
Carbohydrates	7 grams	Calcium	54 mg
Fat	2 grams	Exchanges	½ bread, ½ fat

Whole Grain Nut Bread

12 servings

	Vegetable cooking spray
1	tablespoon wheat germ, divided
½	cup whole wheat flour
½	cup medium rye flour
2	tablespoons cracked wheat flour
2	tablespoons finely chopped walnuts
½	teaspoon baking soda
½	cup buttermilk
1	egg
1	tablespoon dark molasses

Spray 1-quart round casserole with vegetable cooking spray. Sprinkle with 1½ teaspoons wheat germ. Tilt dish to coat. Set aside. In mixing bowl, combine whole wheat flour, rye flour, cracked wheat flour, walnuts, and baking soda. Set aside.

In small mixing bowl, blend buttermilk, egg, and molasses. Add to dry ingredients. (Dough will be sticky.) Spread into prepared casserole, mounding slightly to form round loaf. Sprinkle with 1½ teaspoons wheat germ.

Microwave at 50% (Medium) for 6 to 11 minutes, or until the center springs back when touched lightly, rotating dish after every 3 minutes. Cut into wedges. Serve warm.

Calories	70	Cholesterol	23 mg
Protein	3 grams	Sodium	48 mg
Carbohydrates	10 grams	Calcium	31 mg
Fat	2 grams	Exchanges	1 bread

Naturally Good Treats

30 treats

$\frac{3}{4}$	cup natural no-salt peanut butter
$\frac{1}{4}$	cup honey
3	tablespoons reduced-calorie margarine
$\frac{1}{2}$	cup instant nonfat dry milk powder
$\frac{1}{2}$	cup unsalted sunflower nuts
$\frac{1}{3}$	cup sesame seed
$\frac{1}{3}$	cup cornflake crumbs
$\frac{1}{4}$	cup finely chopped dried apricots
$\frac{2}{3}$	cup flaked coconut

In $1\frac{1}{2}$-quart casserole, combine peanut butter, honey, and margarine. Microwave at High for 1 to 2 minutes, or until hot and mixture can be stirred smooth. Stir in remaining ingredients, except coconut. Shape into 30 balls, about $1\frac{1}{4}$ inches in diameter. Roll each treat in coconut. Chill for at least 3 hours, or until firm.

Calories	86	Cholesterol	—
Protein	3 grams	Sodium	28 mg
Carbohydrates	7 grams	Calcium	20 mg
Fat	7 grams	Exchanges	$\frac{1}{2}$ bread, 1 fat

The following recipes may be prepared on a stove top or in a conventional oven.

Coffee Breakfast Drink

2 servings

¼	cup Quaker Oats (quick or old fashioned, uncooked)
1	cup skim milk
1	teaspoon instant coffee powder
½	teaspoon vanilla
½	teaspoon sugar (optional)
½	cup cracked ice or 4 ice cubes

Place oats in blender container. Blend about 1 minute, stopping blender occasionally to stir oats. Add remaining ingredients; blend on high speed about 1 minute or until smooth.

Calories	85	Cholesterol	2 mg
Protein	6 grams	Sodium	64 mg
Carbohydrates	13 grams	Calcium	159 mg
Fat	1 gram	Exchanges	½ bread, ½ milk

Vegetable Oat Pilaf

8 ½-cup servings

- ½ cup chopped mushrooms
- ½ cup chopped green pepper
- ½ cup sliced green onions
- 2 tablespoons liquid vegetable oil margarine
- 1¾ cups Quaker Oats (quick or old fashioned, uncooked)
- ¼ cup egg substitute or 1 egg
- ¾ cup single strength chicken broth

Saute mushrooms, green pepper, and onions in margarine 2 to 3 minutes. Mix oats and egg substitute until oats are evenly coated. Add oats to vegetable mixture in skillet; cook over medium heat until oats are dry and separated, about 5 to 6 minutes. Add broth; continue cooking 2 to 3 minutes until liquid is absorbed.

Calories	108	Cholesterol	—
Protein	5 grams	Sodium	128 mg
Carbohydrates	13 grams	Calcium	20 mg
Fat	4 grams	Exchanges	½ vegetable, ½ fat, ½ bread

Baked Tuna Loaf with Cucumber Sauce

8 servings

2 $6\frac{1}{2}$ or 7 oz cans tuna packed in water, drained
$\frac{3}{4}$ cup finely chopped celery
$\frac{3}{4}$ cup Quaker Oats (quick or old fashioned, uncooked)
$\frac{1}{2}$ cup skim milk
$\frac{1}{4}$ cup egg substitute or 1 egg
$\frac{1}{8}$ teaspoon pepper
Cucumber sauce (see below)

Heat oven to 350°F. Coat 8 × 4-inch loaf pan with vegetable oil cooking spray or oil lightly. Flake tuna; add remaining ingredients, mixing well. Pat into prepared pan. Bake 40 minutes; let stand 5 minutes before slicing. Serve warm or cold with Cucumber Sauce.

Cucumber Sauce

$1\frac{1}{3}$ cups

1 8 oz container (1 cup) plain yogurt
$\frac{1}{2}$ medium cucumber, finely chopped
2 tablespoons chopped fresh dill or 1 teaspoon dried dill weed
1 teaspoon minced onion

In small bowl, combined all ingredients; mix well. Chill.

Calories	118	Cholesterol	33 mg
Protein	17 grams	Sodium	456 mg
Carbohydrates	8 grams	Calcium	80 mg
Fat	2 grams	Exchanges	1 lean meat, $\frac{1}{2}$ bread, $\frac{1}{4}$ milk, $\frac{1}{8}$ vegetable

Saucy Stuffed Peppers

12 servings

6	medium green peppers
1¼	cups water
2	cups tomato juice
1	6 oz can tomato paste
1	teaspoon oregano leaves, crushed
½	teaspoon garlic powder
½	teaspoon basil leaves, crushed
1	lb lean ground beef
1½	cups Quaker Oats (quick or old fashioned, uncooked)
1	medium tomato, chopped
¼	cup chopped carrot
¼	cup chopped onion

Heat oven to 350° F. Cut peppers in half lengthwise; remove membrane and seeds; set aside. Combine water, 1 cup tomato juice, tomato paste, ½ teaspoon oregano, ¼ teaspoon garlic, and basil. Simmer 10 to 15 minutes.

Combine beef, oats, remaining 1 cup tomato juice, ½ teaspoon oregano, and ¼ teaspoon garlic with tomato, carrot, and onion; mix well. Fill each green pepper halfway with about ⅓ cup meat mixture. Place in 13 × 9-inch glass baking dish; pour sauce evenly over peppers. Bake 45 to 50 minutes.

Calories	155	Cholesterol	34 mg
Protein	16 grams	Sodium	129 mg
Carbohydrates	16 grams	Calcium	32 mg
Fat	3 grams	Exchanges	2 vegetable, 1½ lean meat, ½ bread

Eggplant and Tomato Parmesan

4 servings

1 medium eggplant (about 1 lb)
2 medium tomatoes, chopped
1 6 oz can ($\frac{2}{3}$ cup) low-sodium cocktail vegetable juice
$\frac{1}{2}$ cup Quaker Oats (quick or old fashioned, uncooked)
2 tablespoons minced fresh basil or 1 teaspoon dried basil leaves, crushed
$\frac{1}{4}$ teaspoon oregano leaves, crushed
2 cloves garlic, minced
$\frac{1}{2}$ cup (2 oz) shredded part-skim mozzarella cheese
2 tablespoons grated parmesan cheese

Heat oven to 350°F. Coat 8-inch square glass baking dish or $1\frac{1}{2}$-qt. casserole with vegetable oil cooking spray or oil lightly. Cut eggplant into $\frac{1}{2}$-inch slices. Layer in prepared dish; top with tomatoes. In small bowl, combine remaining ingredients except cheeses. Spread over vegetables; sprinkle evenly with mozzarella cheese, then parmesan cheese. Bake 35 to 40 minutes or until deep golden brown.

Calories	144	Cholesterol	10 mg
Protein	9 grams	Sodium	118 mg
Carbohydrates	18 grams	Calcium	204 mg
Fat	4 grams	Exchanges	2 vegetables, $\frac{1}{2}$ bread, 1 lean meat

Crunchy Apple Crisp

4 servings

4 cups peeled sliced apples
¼ cup water or apple juice
4 teaspoons brown sugar substitute or firmly packed brown sugar
2 teaspoons lemon juice
¾ teaspoon cinnamon
½ cup Quaker Oats (quick or old fashioned, uncooked)
2 tablespoons chopped walnuts
1 tablespoon brown sugar substitute or packed brown sugar
1 tablespoon soft vegetable oil margarine

Combine apples, water, brown sugar substitute, lemon juice, and cinnamon; toss lightly to coat apples. Layer on bottom of 8-inch square glass baking dish.

Heat oven to 375°F. Combine oats, nuts, and brown sugar substitute. Add margarine; mix well. Sprinkle over apples. Bake about 30 minutes or until apples are tender and topping is lightly browned. Serve warm or chilled.

Calories	158	Cholesterol	—
Protein	2 grams	Sodium	40 mg
Carbohydrates	24 grams	Calcium	19 mg
Fat	6 grams	Exchanges	1 fat, 1 fruit, ¾ bread

Chicken Cutlets Supreme

6 servings

- 3/4 cup Ground Oat Flour
- 1 tablespoon snipped fresh dill or 1 teaspoon dried dill weed
- 1/8 teaspoon lemon pepper
- 1/4 cup egg substitute or 1 egg
- 1/4 cup water
- 3 chicken breasts, boned, skinned, and split
- 2 tablespoons soft vegetable oil margarine, melted

Heat oven to 375°F. Spray 13 × 9-inch baking pan with vegetable oil cooking spray or oil lightly. In shallow dish, combine Ground Oat Flour, dill, and lemon pepper. In another shallow dish, combine egg substitute and water. Lightly pound chicken to even thickness between sheets of plastic wrap or wax paper. Coat with dry ingredients; shake off excess. Dip into egg mixture, then coat again with dry ingredients. Place in prepared pan. Drizzle margarine evenly over chicken. Bake 35 minutes.

Ground Oat Flour

3/4 cup

Place 1 cup Quaker Oats (quick or old fashioned, uncooked) in blender or food processor. Cover; blend about 1 minute, stopping blender occasionally to stir oats.

Calories	208	Cholesterol	59 mg
Protein	25 grams	Sodium	112 mg
Carbohydrates	9 grams	Calcium	28 mg
Fat	8 grams	Exchanges	3/4 bread, 3 lean meat, 3/4 fat

Turkey Cranberry Cutlets

4 servings

1	medium orange, cut in half
1	cup fresh or frozen cranberries
¼	cup sugar
1	teaspoon grated orange peel
1	cup Quaker Oats (quick or old fashioned, uncooked)
2	tablespoons minced parsley
½	teaspoon poultry seasoning
1	lb fresh turkey breast slices
3	tablespoons vegetable oil

Juice one half of orange; set aside. Scoop out pulp from remaining orange half. Place cranberries, orange pulp, orange peel, and sugar in blender or food processor. Blend on medium speed about 30 seconds or until mixture is coarsely chopped.

Combine oats and seasonings in blender or food processor; cover. Blend about 1 minute stopping occasionally to stir. Dip each turkey slice in reserved orange juice; coat with oat mixture. Saute in oil over medium heat about 2 to 3 minutes on each side, or until evenly browned and tender. Serve with sauce.

Calories	380	Cholesterol	70 mg
Protein	31 grams	Sodium	80 mg
Carbohydrates	36 grams	Calcium	60 mg
Fat	14 grams	Exchanges	4 lean meat, 2 fruit, ½ starch/bread

Garden Style Pizza

8 servings

- 1¼ cups all-purpose flour
- ¾ cup Ground Oat Flour (see p. 206)
- 1 teaspoon baking powder
- ½ teaspoon salt (optional)
- ⅔ cup skim milk
- ¼ cup vegetable oil
- 2 cups sliced mushrooms
- 1½ cups shredded carrots
- 1 cup thinly sliced zucchini
- ½ cup chopped onion
- 2 tablespoons soft vegetable oil margarine
- 1 8 oz can pizza sauce
- 2 cups (8 oz.) shredded part-skim mozzarella cheese
- ½ teaspoon Italian seasoning

Heat oven to 425°F. Spray 14-inch round pizza pan or 15 × 10-inch jelly roll pan with vegetable oil cooking spray or oil lightly. Combine flour, oat flour, baking powder, and salt. Add milk and oil; stir with fork until mixture forms a ball. Knead dough on lightly floured surface about 10 times. With greased fingers, press dough into prepared pan; shape edge to form rim. Bake about 15 minutes.

Saute mushrooms, carrots, zucchini, and onion in margarine over medium heat about 3 minutes. Spoon pizza sauce over partially baked crust, spreading evenly to edge; top with sauted vegetables. Sprinkle with cheese and Italian seasoning; continue baking about 15 minutes or until cheese is melted.

Calories	330	Cholesterol	17 mg
Protein	13 grams	Sodium	395 mg
Carbohydrates	29 grams	Calcium	247 mg
Fat	18 grams	Exchanges	1½ bread, 1½ lean meat, 2 fat, 2½ vegetable

Stuffed Sole

8 servings

1	10 oz pkg. frozen chopped spinach
1	cup sliced mushrooms
½	cup sliced green onions
2	tablespoons soft vegetable oil margarine
1¾	cups Quaker Oats (quick or old fashioned, uncooked)
¼	cup egg substitute or 1 egg
1	teaspoon salt (optional)
¼	cup lemon juice
8	sole or flounder fillets (about 2 lb)
	Paprika

Thaw spinach, reserving liquid. Heat oven to 375°F. Saute mushrooms and onions in margarine over medium heat 3 to 4 minutes. Add oats, egg substitute, salt, 2 tablespoons lemon juice, reserved spinach, and liquid; mix well. Divide spinach mixture evenly among fillets, spreading to within ½-inch of edges. Roll up; place seam side down in 13 × 9-inch glass baking dish. Sprinkle with remaining 2 tablespoons lemon juice; dust with paprika. Bake 25 minutes or until fish flakes easily with fork.

Calories	333	Cholesterol	101 mg
Protein	39 grams	Sodium	163 mg
Carbohydrates	15 grams	Calcium	79 mg
Fat	13 grams	Exchanges	4 lean meat, 1 vegetable, 1 bread

Italian Zucchini Bake

8 servings

3	cups shredded zucchini
1/2	cup chopped onion
1	tablespoon vegetable oil
1 1/4	cups Quaker Oats (quick or old fashioned, uncooked)
1/4	cup (1 oz) shredded part-skim mozzarella cheese
1/4	cup egg substitute or 1 egg
1/2	teaspoon basil or oregano leaves, crushed
1/2	teaspoon salt (optional)
1/8	teaspoon pepper
1/3	cup tomato sauce

Heat oven to 375°F. Coat 8-inch square glass baking dish with vegetable oil cooking spray or oil lightly. Press zucchini between paper towels to remove excess moisture. Saute onion in oil until tender; transfer to large bowl. Add zucchini and remaining ingredients except tomato sauce; mix well. Spread into prepared baking dish. Spread tomato sauce evenly over top. Bake 30 minutes or until heated through.

Calories	104	Cholesterol	2 mg
Protein	5 grams	Sodium	85 mg
Carbohydrates	12 grams	Calcium	54 mg
Fat	4 grams	Exchanges	1 vegetable, 3/4 bread, 1/4 lean meat, 1/2 fat

Very Blueberry Muffins

1 dozen muffins

- 1⅓ cups all-purpose flour
- 1 cup Quaker Oats (quick or old fashioned, uncooked)
- ¼ cup brown sugar substitute or firmly packed brown sugar
- 1 tablespoon baking powder
- ½ teaspoon salt (optional)
- ½ teaspoon cinnamon
- 1 cup skim milk
- ¼ egg substitute, or 1 egg
- 3 tablespoons vegetable oil
- 1 cup fresh or frozen blueberries

Heat oven to 425°F. Spray 12 medium muffin cups with vegetable oil cooking spray or line with paper baking cups. Combine dry ingredients. Add milk, egg substitute, and oil; stir just until dry ingredients are moistened. Fold in blueberries; fill prepared muffin cups ⅔ full. Bake 25 to 30 minutes or until light golden brown.

Calories	124	Cholesterol	—
Protein	4 grams	Sodium	122 mg
Carbohydrates	18 grams	Calcium	53 mg
Fat	4 grams	Exchanges	1 bread, 1 fat, ½ fruit

Oat Pancakes

12 pancakes

1 cup all-purpose flour
½ cup Quaker Oats (quick or old fashioned, uncooked)
1 tablespoon baking powder
½ teaspoon salt (optional)
1 cup skim milk
¼ cup egg substitute or 1 egg, beaten
2 tablespoons vegetable oil

Head griddle over medium-high heat (or preheat electric griddle or skillet to 375°F). Oil lightly. Combine dry ingredients. Add milk, egg substitute, and oil; stir just until dry ingredients are moistened. For each pancake, pour about ¼ cup batter on hot griddle. Turn when tops are covered with bubbles and edges look cooked. Turn only once.

Calories	236	Cholesterol	1 mg
Protein	8 grams	Sodium	361 mg
Carbohydrates	33 grams	Calcium	147 mg
Fat	8 grams	Exchanges	2 bread, 1½ fat, ½ milk

15

The Wellness Buying Guide

In this chapter we will address the question of how to buy the Wellness way at the grocery store. Do you face confusion at the grocery store and ask yourself, "What is good for me to eat and what isn't?" This chapter will help you through that confusion. The key to Wellness buying is *reading the label* and determining how much fat and simple sugars are in the food product you intend to buy. Handy tips are also provided, for example, on which types of oil to buy and which types to avoid.

Each of the following sections is divided into specific food types. Each discusses the mechanics of wise food selection and, in some sections, includes foods to be avoided. This chapter will be very helpful in planning your shopping list and will assist you in educating yourself about Wellness buying.

BEVERAGES

Water should be your beverage of choice. Other beverages that are low in fat are fruit and vegetable juices and low fat or skim milk. Coffee is also an acceptable alternative—it contains no calories at all.

To determine whether or not a beverage is low in fat, read the label. It should read 2 grams of fat or less per an 8-ounce serving.

BREADS

Some breads contain no fat at all. These include French or Italian breads, pita bread, soft nonfried tortillas, and bagels. Hard rolls also contain no fat. Low fat breads include English muffins, sandwich bread or toast, pan rolls, bread sticks, and cracker meal. Examples of high fat breads and thus breads to be avoided are sourdough and biscuits. Also, when making pancakes or waffles, choose the mixes to which you add the oil or water. That way, no extra fat has to be used for cooking.

CEREALS AND CRACKERS

Almost all types of cooked and dry cereals contain little to no fat. Most crackers are made with animal or vegetable fat. Try to choose crackers with no added fat or those made only with a little fat. To determine the fat content, read the label and choose the crackers made with 3 grams of fat or less per 1-ounce serving.

Some examples of these crackers include melba toast, Ry-Krisp, pretzels, and oyster crackers. Potato and tortilla chips can be very high in fat. Choose only those fried in the acceptable oils listed later in the chapter.

CHEESE

Most cheeses are very high in fat. Seventy percent of the calories in cheese comes from fat, so be very careful when buying cheeses. Some low fat cheeses are farmer cheese, pot cheese, and ricotta cheese made with part skim milk. Low fat cottage cheese and the new "lighter" cheeses are acceptable, but read the label.

COFFEE CREAMER

This is a hidden source of fat for a lot of people. Most powdered creamers are very high in saturated fat, and are typically made with coconut or palm oil—the worst nonmeat fats. Avoid them. Suitable alternatives are skim or evaporated skim milk. Low fat mild or instant nonfat dry milk can also be used to lighten up your coffee.

MILK

The best milk is skim or 1 percent milk. Buttermilk is also a low fat milk choice.

YOGURT

Read the label on the yogurt carton and choose one with 2 to 3 grams of fat or less per 8-ounce serving.

DESSERTS AND SWEETS

Cakes: Most cakes are made with animal or saturated vegetable fat, and are, therefore, very high in fat. Choose a cake mix that contains little or no fat and add your own safflower or sunflower oil. Read the label on the cake mix and choose a mix with 4 grams or less of fat per serving. The best cakes are angel food and homemade low fat cakes.

Candy: Candy usually contains little fat but a lot of calories. I would recommend staying away from it, unless it is the sugar-free type. However, even sugar-free candy can contain a lot of calories. Some sugar-free candy contains calories from carob and fructose, which, though different forms of sugar, are no more healthy than simple sugars. Read the label to check the calorie content.

Cookies: Most cookies are made with animal or saturated vegetable fats. Choose a cookie that has 3 grams or less of fat per 1 ounce serving. Low fat cookies include animal crackers, ginger snaps, fig bars, graham crackers, and molasses cookies.

Frozen Desserts: Sorry, no ice cream. Frozen dairy desserts that are acceptable are fruit ices, frozen fruit juice, sherbet, low-fat frozen yogurt, sugar-free popsicles, fudgesicles, and the diet frozen desserts. Ice milk is also an acceptable frozen dessert.

FATS AND OILS

The best margarines are those that are low in saturated fat and high in polyunsaturated fat. The very best are the new liquid margarines. Read the label and choose the margarine that contains twice as much polyunsaturated fat as saturated fat. The best oils are safflower, sunflower, and corn oil.

FISH, POULTRY, AND LEAN MEATS

Choose plain or unprocessed fish, shellfish, and poultry. These are the leanest. Lean meats are those with the least visible fat. Lean cuts of beef are from the flank, sirloin, chuck, and rump roast. Lamb is lean, but trim off all the visible fat. Some pork cuts, such as loin chops, tenderloin, and rib chops, are lean. All cuts of veal are acceptable when the fat is trimmed completely.

If you are going to use a processed meat, choose one with 3 grams or less of fat per ounce. When you eat poultry, remove the skin.

FRUIT

All fresh or canned fruit is acceptable in terms of fat. However, be careful with canned fruits because they commonly contain a lot of sugar and calories. Choose fruit canned in fruit juice, light syrup, or water.

MAIN DISHES

Canned Foods and Frozen Foods: Read the label and choose canned foods which contain 10 grams or less of fat per 2 cups. For frozen dinners choose the ones containing less than 10 grams of fat per dinner. If you are preparing a packaged meat, fish, or poultry main dish, choose the ones with 10 grams or less of fat per 2 cups and don't add additional oil or margarine. If the main dish requires that you add the meat, poultry, or fish, choose ones with 1 gram or less of fat.

Low fat canned foods are chow mein, chop suey, meatless spaghetti sauce, tuna and noodles, and vegetable stew.

Low fat frozen dinners include chow mein and chop suey of all types, sliced chicken and chicken and noodles, and baked fish. Turkey frozen dinners are also low in fat.

Packaged main dishes to choose are oriental main dish mixes, pizza mix without meat, meatless spaghetti, and tuna main dish mixes without cheese or cream as main ingredients.

Meat Substitutes: Remember that you must combine meatless proteins to supply all the essential amino acids your body needs. Therefore, if you eat no meat, fish, or fowl, you must eat a combination of the following on a daily basis: legumes (beans, peas, and lentils) and low fat dairy products, or legumes and bread, cereal, or grain products and low fat dairy products, nuts and seeds and low fat dairy products. Tofu also supplies a no fat source of protein and supplies almost all of the essential amino acids by itself.

Examples of low fat meat substitutes are beans prepared without fat or meat, or lentils and peas prepared without fat or meat.

Nuts and Seeds: Nuts are relatively high in fat, but some nuts are worse than others. Avoid coconut and nuts roasted in coconut or palm oil. While seeds and nuts are good sources of protein, they are also concentrated sources of calories, 80 percent of which comes from fat. Therefore, be very careful with the number of nuts you eat.

Nuts that are lowest in fat are walnuts, pine nuts, beechnuts, pecans, chestnuts, and almonds. Nuts higher in fat are filberts, peanuts and peanut butter, cashews and cashew butter, and pistachio and macadamia nuts. All seeds are acceptable but be cautious and make sure they are not roasted in coconut oil.

Pasta, Noodles, and Rice: Plain pasta, noodles, and rice are low in saturated fat and cholesterol, with the exception of egg noodles. Read the label and make sure that they have 1 gram or less of fat per ½ cup without added ingredients.

SALAD DRESSINGS

Read the label when buying salad dressings, and buy those with minimal amounts of cream, cheese, and egg yolk. The best salad dressing is lemon juice or vinegar and oil, made with very little oil. Use low calorie mayonnaise or bottled dressing. Watch out for horseradish sauce made with cream or mayonnaise.

SOUPS

Many commercial soups are low in fat when prepared with acceptable ingredients such as skim milk. Choose soups with 3 grams of fat or less per cup without added ingredients. Examples of such soups include bouillon, broth, beef noodle and vegetable, bean, chicken noodle and vegetable and rice, Manhattan-style clam chowder, lentil, minestrone, pea (without bacon), tomato, turkey noodle and vegetable, vegetable and vegetable beef, and chicken or turkey.

VEGETABLES

All canned, fresh, or frozen vegetables are low in fat.

USING FOOD LABELS

Food labels can be very helpful when eating the Wellness way. Remember we mentioned earlier that food labels list ingredients from the highest to lowest amount contained, in descending order. In other words, the ingredient that makes up the largest amount of the product is listed first, the next largest is listed second, and so on. Therefore, you know what you are buying and eating by reading the label.

Some acceptable ingredients are carob powder, cocoa, corn oil, cottonseed oil, diglycerides, hydrolyzed (added hydrogen) ingredients, monoglycerides (unsaturated fats), nonfat dry milk, safflower oil, sesame oil, skim milk, soybean oil, and sunflower oil.

Unacceptable ingredients, because of their fat content, are bacon fat, beef fat, butter, chicken fat, chocolate (real and imitation), cocoa butter, coconut and coconut oil, cream and cream sauce, egg and egg-yolk solids, hardened fat or oil, hydrogenated fat or oil, lard, meat fat, milk chocolate, palm or palm kernel oil, pork fat, shortening, turkey fat, vegetable shortening, and whole-milk solids.

A WORD ABOUT SALT

Many people have problems with their blood pressure. Therefore, they need to be concerned with how much salt they eat. The lower your salt intake, the better off you are in terms of blood pressure control. Food labels can be a great help in keeping salt intake to a minimum. High sodium (salt) ingredients are salt (sodium chloride), monosodium glutamate, brine (salt water), broth, bouillon, baking soda (sodium bicarbonate), baking powder, and soy sauce.

WATCH OUT FOR SUGAR

Sugar, like salt, can be disguised in a number of ways. Read the label and avoid these sources of sugar: sucrose, fructose, dextrose, corn syrup, invert sugar, honey, molasses, maple syrup, and brown sugar.

As you can see, buying food in a Wellness way is not an impossibility. Learning which foods are to be avoided or included is a matter of reading the labels and applying the knowledge that you have acquired about the content of the foods in terms of fats, sugars, proteins, carbohydrates, and calories.

16

Dining Out the Wellness Way

America loves to eat out. We are a society on the move, and being on the go cuts into the time available for meal preparation. Consequently, we eat out often. In fact, some studies have shown that we eat one out of every three meals out of our homes.

You might believe that because you eat out so much, it is impossible to lose weight. This chapter will help you to eat in the Wellness way when you eat out. It contains tips on how to order at a restaurant, definitions of some terms commonly used in restaurant menus, and what to ask the waiter in reference to these categories. Finally, we will discuss the different types of restaurants and the variety of foods each type serves.

THOUGHTS ON EATING OUT

When you sit down in a restaurant, remember that you are the boss. The restaurant is there to serve you and to please you, so don't be intimidated. Order what you want and remember that you are usually not limited by what is on the menu. For example, if you want the sauce to be left off the fish that you ordered, ask it to be served on the side or not at all. If you prefer your fish or other grilled meat to be grilled without butter, ask the waiter to inform the chef of your preference. If you would like to order smaller portions, order from the appetizer menu as your main course.

If it is not noted on the menu, ask how a selection is prepared. If the menu says "sauteed," ask if the item is sauteed in butter, oil, lard, or margarine, or simply request that your choice be sauteed in a reduced amount of vegetable oil. Ask the waiter if margarine can be served in place of butter and if skim milk could be substituted for whole milk. Ask if a dish can be prepared with vegetable oil rather than animal fat or butter. Ask that the chef trim all the visible fat off your cut of meat. If you are eating poultry, ask the chef to remove the skin. If the poultry is served with the skin on, remove it yourself.

Request that your foods be broiled, baked, or steamed rather than deep fat fried or sauteed. If you want dessert, request fresh fruit or canned fruit in a light syrup. Remember, if you make these requests in a pleasant but firm manner you will be able to maintain your Wellness diet and enjoy eating out with your friends.

Breakfast

When eating breakfast in a restaurant, there are many ways to eat in a Wellness way. Choose fresh fruit or a glass of juice. Ask that your bread, bagel, or English muffin be toasted dry and that margarine be served on the side. Hot cereals are low in fat and sugar and are wise choices. Use skim or 1 percent fat milk on your cereal. Quiche, omelettes, and other egg-based dishes are typically high in fat and often omelettes are made with butter. You can request a "yolk-free" omelette, but omit the cheese. A waffle or pancake (made without oil) would be a good breakfast item as well.

Beverages

Alcohol adds calories. There is no fat in alcohol but there are calories. So if you drink alcohol, be sure to include it in your calorie count. Other beverage choices include seltzer, diet sodas, fruit juices, and, of course, water.

Appetizers

Appetizers are often loaded with fat so choose carefully. Steamed seafood, raw vegetables, and fresh fruit are low fat appetizers. Some people order deep-fried vegetables, thinking that the fact that they are eating vegetables means that they are eating a Wellness food. However, the breading and oil in deep-fried vegetables overshadow the benefit of the vegetables themselves.

Entrees

Simplicity in food preparation usually means that the food is low in fat. Avoid casseroles and foods with heavy sauces. Poultry and fish prepared in a simple manner are your best choices. Be careful because even broiled items are sometimes broiled in their own fat—so ask the waiter if the chef can dry-broil your selection. An alternative to dry-broiling is using lemon during the broiling process.

SALADS

Salads are an excellent Wellness food. They offer bulk, flavor, and variety to your menu. Fresh greens and vegetables tossed together can be eaten either as a meal by itself or as an accompaniment to an entree. A word of caution is necessary, however, when ordering salads. If you load your salad with cheese, meats, or oily croutons, you are not doing yourself a favor. These are all fatty foods and transform your Wellness salad into a fatty food. Also, be cautious when it comes to salad dressings. All creamy dressings are high in fat and many colored dressings, like French, are high in sugar. Use lemon juice or vinegar with a small amount of oil in a four to one ratio as your salad dressing instead of those other high fat/high sugar dressings. Also, many restaurants offer low calorie dressings for their salads.

SIDE DISHES

Side dishes are good compliments to your meal if they are low fat or fat free. Baked potatoes or steamed green vegetables are excellent accompaniments to your meal. Avoid fried foods or those that are doused in butter. Try yogurt, lemon juice, or a low fat salad dressing as sauces on your vegetables or potatoes.

LOW FAT FOOD SELECTIONS

Many descriptions of a food selection on a menu can tip you off that the item is a low fat preparation. "Dry-broiled" means that no sauce or butter is used in the broiling process. "In its own juice" generally means an item has been cooked in its own juice as opposed to being cooked in a high fat sauce or oil, but be careful that "in its own juice" doesn't mean it was cooked in its own fat. Broiled and roasted foods are usually cooked without the addition of sauces or oils, but this can vary, so ask. "Poached" items are generally low fat items, as are steamed and roasted items. Other commonly low fat foods are those that are "pickled," "in cocktail sauce," "smoked," "in broth," or "in a tomato base." However, these items also can be high in salt. Therefore, if you have a blood pressure problem and need to restrict your salt intake, avoid these items.

High Fat Foods

Menu items that are typically high in fat and therefore should be avoided are those that are "buttered," "buttery," or "in butter sauce." Also high in fat are foods that are "sauteed," "pan-fried," "crispy," "fried," or "braised." Those foods that are "creamed" or "in cream sauce" are generally very high in fat content. Cheese sauces, whether "au gratin," "parmesan," or "escalloped," really add to the fat content of food. "Hollandaise sauce" is almost pure fat.

ETHNIC RESTAURANTS AND THE FOODS THEY SERVE

Chinese

Chinese food is a delicious choice that also contains Wellness food. However, a few tips are necessary to help you make wise decisions when ordering Chinese cuisine. Skip the noodles. Often they are fatty and only add calories without contributing to the taste of the food. Choose dishes that are boiled, steamed, or lightly stir-fried. Examples are stir-fried chicken or vegetables. Ask that your dish be stir-fried in vegetable oil, rather than sauteed. Wonton soup is low in fat, as is hot and sour soup. The salt content of Chinese food can be very high, so request that soy sauce be served on the side and that the MSG be left out. Egg foo young and dishes prepared with lobster sauce are high in fat because egg yolks are used, so avoid these foods. Hunan- and Szechuan-style food is usually high in calories because the meat or poultry is usually fried first in hot oil. Avoid all the dishes that are deep-fried such as sweet and sour dishes. Eat the steamed rice.

French

Simplicity is the key to low fat French food. Watch out for French onion soup—it is loaded with fat and calories. Sauces are the heart of classic French cuisine, but be wary. Hollandaise, bechamel, and bernaise sauces are all high in fat because they are made with eggs and butter. Alternatives are bordelaise and nouvelle sauces, which are lighter. But these sauces may still be made of cream, so ask the waiter or waitress. Order the sauces on the side and only use a small amount for the taste. Avoid au gratin dishes as they are very high in fat. Order simply prepared lean meat, fish, fowl, and vegetables. The less sauce the better.

Greek

The key to eating Greek food in a Wellness way is to seek foods that are prepared in a minimal amount of oil. Tzatziki is an appetizer made with yogurt and cucumbers and is very low fat. Pita bread is a low fat bread and Greek salads are low in fat. The cheese used, feta, is slightly lower in fat than hard cheeses. For your main entree choose plaki, fish that has been cooked in tomatoes, onions, and garlic; or a spit-broiled shish-ka-bob. Be wary and avoid phyllo dough, which is very high in fat, and babaganoosh, an eggplant appetizer prepared with fat.

Indian

Indian food is generally low in fat. Skip the appetizers since they are fried in oil, and have a plain salad instead. Many Indian dishes use yogurt as a base and creatively use spices to add flavor. Tandoori chicken and fish dishes are excellent low fat choices as these foods are marinated in spices and then roasted in a clay pot. Be sure to request the chef to avoid using butter as a basting sauce for your Tandoori food item. Shish kabob is lamb broiled over coals and is a good choice if lean lamb is used. Be sure to request the chef to avoid using ghee, clarified butter, in the preparation of vegetables. Curried dishes are good if the base (the meat or fowl) is lean.

Italian

Italian foods always bring to mind pasta. Pasta is an excellent Wellness food as long as it is not filled with cheese or fatty meat or tossed with butter. As a sauce, choose red or white clam sauce and avoid cream sauces or meat sauces. Marsala and marinara sauces are good choices. Pasta primavera prepared with a reduced amount of oil is an excellent low fat food selection. Avoid dishes like scallopine or parmigiana, since they are usually prepared by adding fats. Eating a low fat entree such as veal prepared without heavy sauces and having pasta on the side is an excellent Wellness choice.

Japanese

Japanese foods are excellent Wellness foods. Pickled vegetables are low in fat and calories and sashimi and sushi are also very low in fat. Be sure that you choose a Japanese restaurant that has not had trouble with fish contaminated by parasites. Deep-fried dishes like tempura should be avoided. As with most sauces, ask that yours be served on the side. Good low fat Japanese food choices are nabemono, chicken teriyaki, and menfui. Look for the word "yadimono," which means broiled.

Mexican

Mexican food, because of its high cheese content, is usually avoided by dieters. However, there are some foods which are acceptable. Choose tortillas made with corn and then baked, not the deep-fried flour tortillas. Load up the baked tortillas with salsa and guacamole as appetizers, but don't eat too much guacamole; it is made from avocados, which are high in fat. Mexican salads with lemon squeezed over the top are very good. Cerviche, marinated fish, is very low in fat. Choose chicken or shrimp tostadas made with corn tortillas (not fried) as a main course. Avoid the refried beans because they are usually cooked in lard. Ask that the cheese and sour cream garnishes be left off or served on the side.

FAST-FOOD WELLNESS

Americans are always in a hurry, and I am no exception. Chances are good that you are no exception either. That is why the fast-food industry has become a multimillion-dollar business—it caters to the needs of Americans in a hurry. Think of fast foods and you conjure up the image of greasy french fries and fatty hamburgers. Well, you're right; most fast food is primarily fatty and greasy food. But there is also a lot of fast food that is Wellness food—food you can eat while on the Wellness diet, and food that will aid you in weight loss as well as weight maintenance.

This chapter includes a listing of many restaurants and the variety of foods that are available, to aid you in choosing Wellness foods. Next to each food item you will be given the calorie, carbohydrate, protein, and fat content of that food. Following that entry are the exchanges which each food represents on the Wellness diet.

Also found on these fast-food lists are the values for fast foods not usually thought of as Wellness foods. I have included these for two reasons. First, to provide you with information to educate yourself about the content of certain foods. For instance, did you have any idea that a fish sandwich from a fast-food restaurant has as much fat as a hamburger? Many people think that because they are eating fish they are cutting down on their fat. However, fish sandwiches contain breaded fish and are deep-fried, both of which add significantly to their fat content.

With the listing of all foods that are commonly available in fast-food restaurants, you can evaluate the foods you have been eating. After this evaluation you will be able to appraise just how much of a positive change will take place by following the

Wellness diet. If you find that you have been eating many grams of saturated fat on a daily basis, and you change your eating habits to include relatively few, doing so will give you a sense of accomplishment as well as result in significant weight loss.

The second reason to include values for foods served in fast-food restaurants that aren't considered Wellness foods is because of human nature. There will be times when you crave a certain food. I know that sometimes I have an overwhelming desire for french fries. I put it off and put it off, but eventually I just have to eat some french fries—and not just the small-size serving either. Occasionally you too will give in to your cravings. But when you do, you can evaluate the impact on your diet and continue from there. You will find that an occasional trailing off the diet will not have a major impact. In fact it is important not to fall into the trap of thinking, "Well, I binged just now. I might as well binge the rest of the day," and eat a double cheeseburger with your french fries. Accept the fact that you binged and continue on the diet.

By using this list you can visit these fast-food restaurants when you are in a hurry, or just too tired to cook, and you will *not* sabotage your weight loss efforts. You will be able to maintain your weight loss program by choosing Wellness foods.

For instance, when I am in a hurry, I go through Wendy's or Rax, buy a plain potato, and top it with diet Italian dressing. Voila! A low fat, high carbohydrate meal that also contains some fiber. Salads and low calorie dressings are also usually available.

I am very fond of fast-food salad bars where there is usually an array of fresh fruits and vegetables. Often, soft flour tortillas (not fried) are available which are a nice change of pace to accompany a trip to the salad bar.

Be careful, though. Stay away from the high-calorie salad dressings and the potato and pasta salads. In restaurants these are typically very high in fat because a lot of mayonnaise is added to them.

This chapter demonstrates that living on a Wellness diet does not mean you can't go out to eat with your friends at restaurants they like. There will always be something you can eat and enjoy.

Exchange Equivalents of Selected Fast-Food Restaurants

	Calories	Carbohydrate	Protein	Fat
ARBY'S				
Beef 'n Cheddar sandwich	490	51	24	21
Chicken Club sandwich	621	57	26	32
Ham 'n Cheese sandwich	353	33	26	13
Junior roast beef sandwich	218	22	12	8
Regular roast beef sandwich	353	32	22	15
Super roast beef sandwich	501	50	25	22
Turkey deluxe sandwich	510	46	28	24
BURGER CHEF				
Hamburger	250	23	12	12
Cheeseburger	304	24	14	17
Double hamburger	325	28	20	15
Double cheeseburger	434	24	24	26
Big Chef	535	41	25	30
Super Chef	600	39	29	37
Skipper's Treat	604	39	29	37
Rancher Platter	640	44	30	38
Mariner Platter	680	85	32	24

Continued

	Calories	Carbohydrate	Protein	Fat
BURGER CHEF (*cont.*)				
French fries	187	25	3	9
Milk shake, chocolate	310	48	9	9
BURGER KING				
Hamburger	290	29	15	13
Cheeseburger	350	30	18	17
Double hamburger	420	30	25	22
Double cheeseburger	530	32	30	31
Whopper	630	50	26	36
Double Beef Whopper	850	52	44	52
Whopper with cheese	740	52	32	45
Double Whopper with cheese	950	54	50	60
Whopper Jr.	370	31	15	20
Whopper Jr. with cheese	420	32	18	25
Whaler	488	45	19	27
Whaler with cheese	530	46	21	30
Onion rings	274	28	4	16
French fries	227	24	3	13
Milk shake, chocolate	374	60	8	11
DAIRY QUEEN				
Double hamburger	530	33	36	28
Hamburger	360	33	21	16
Hamburger with cheese	410	33	24	20
Brazier Cheese Dog	580	45	22	34
Brazier Chili Dog	570	47	21	32
Brazier Dog	520	44	17	27
Brazier french fries, small	200	25	2	10

	Calories	Carbohydrate	Protein	Fat
DAIRY QUEEN (*cont.*)				
Onion rings	280	31	4	16
D.Q. Chocolate dipped cone, small	190	25	3	9
D.Q. cone, small	140	22	3	4
Fish sandwich	400	41	20	17
Fish sandwich with cheese	440	39	24	21
FRIENDLY ICE CREAM				
Big Burger	420	33	36	15
Big Burger with cheese	480	34	40	19
Bounty burger	570	40	37	28
Coleslaw	80	6	1	7
Cake cone (reg. 4 oz)	260	31	5	13
Sugar cone (reg. 4 oz)	300	40	5	14
Fish	340	31	14	17
French fries	125	16	2	6
Ham and cheese	400	26	20	24
Hamburger	260	29	18	7
KENTUCKY FRIED CHICKEN				
Original recipe drumstick	147	3	14	9
Original recipe breast	276	10	20	17
Original recipe thigh	278	8	18	19
Original recipe wing	181	6	12	12
Extra crispy drumstick	173	6	13	11
Extra crispy thigh	371	14	20	26
Extra crispy wing	218	8	12	16
Extra crispy breast	354	17	18	24
Mashed potatoes	59	12	2	1

Continued

	Calories	Carbohydrate	Protein	Fat
KENTUCKY FRIED CHICKEN (*cont.*)				
Coleslaw	105	12	1	6
Biscuit	269	32	4	14
LONG JOHN SILVER'S				
Breaded clams, 1 order	526	58	17	31
Breaded oysters, 1 piece	60	6	2	3
Chicken planks, 1 piece	152	10	9	8
Coleslaw (4 oz)	182	11	1	15
Corn-on-the-cob	176	29	5	4
Fish with batter, 1 piece	202	11	13	12
Fish and fries, 3 pieces	853	64	43	48
French fries (3 oz.)	247	31	4	12
Hush Puppies, 2 pieces	145	18	3	7
Ocean scallops, dinner	747	66	17	45
Batter fried shrimp dinner	711	60	17	45
3-piece dinner (includes fish, chips, and coleslaw)	1180	93	47	70
MCDONALD'S				
Hamburger	263	28	12	11
Cheeseburger	318	29	15	16
Quarter Pounder	427	29	25	24
Quarter Pounder with cheese	525	31	30	32
Big Mac	570	39	25	35
Filet-o-Fish, with sauce	435	36	15	26
French fries, regular	220	26	3	12
Egg McMuffin	340	31	19	16

	Cal-ories	Carbo-hydrate	Protein	Fat
McDONALD'S (*cont.*)				
Pork sausage	210	1	10	19
Scrambled eggs	180	3	13	13
Shake, vanilla	352	60	9	39
English muffin, buttered	186	30	5	5
PIZZA HUT				
1 slice medium pizza, thin crust	180	22.5	10	
Standard with cheese				5.5
Standard with pepperoni	202	22.5	10	8
Standard with pork and mushrooms	196	20	11	8
DOMINO'S PIZZA				
12″ cheese pizza, 2 slices	340	52	18	6
12″ pepperoni pizza, 2 slices	380	48	20	12
16″ cheese pizza, 2 slices	400	58	24	8
16″ pepperoni pizza, 2 slices	440	56	24	14
WENDY'S				
Cheeseburger				
Single Cheese	420	27	25	52
Double Cheese	630	24	45	57

Continued

	Cal-ories	Carbo-hydrate	Protein	Fat
WENDY'S (*cont.*)				
Triple Cheese	1040	35	72	68
Chili	260	26	21	8
French fries	280	35	4	14
Frosty	390	54	9	16
Hamburger				
Single	350	27	21	18
Double	560	24	41	34

Source: Reprinted with permission from Michael Jackson and Sarah Fitschner, *Fast Food Guide* (Washington, DC: Workman, 1986). Copyright 1986, Center for Science in the Public Interest.

17

Food Values

This chapter of The Wellness Way to Weight Loss is devoted to listing foods and their corresponding values. The values listed are for calories (Kcal) contained in the portion of food and for the amount of protein (Pro), carbohydrate (Cho), fat (Fat), saturated fat (Sfa), and dietary fiber (Dfib). These foods are listed in portions that are commonly served. For example, the values listed for cottage cheese are for ½ cup of cottage cheese.

I felt that this was an appropriate subject for this late in the book because it will help you in determining what foods are Wellness foods and what foods you should avoid. This chapter will enable you to look up the values for the many different foods that you eat. Looking up the values for foods is an educational process, and undoubtedly you will encounter a few surprises. I am sure that some foods you thought were high in either protein, fat, or carbohydrates are not, and other foods that you had preconceived ideas about actually have different values than you anticipated. You can find out how much fat is in a food and how much of the fat is saturated.

Foods are grouped according to food type, and are identified on the basis of the food's name, the brand name (where applicable), and the portion size. Values are given in grams.

Note that a blank space does not mean that the value of a food is zero. Rather, the space indicates that the data was not available. Protein, carbohydrates, fat, saturated fat, and dietary fiber are all listed in gram measurements. Also note that while this listing is extensive, it is by no means complete. There are many books available which have more extensive listings. Refer to the bibliography for some of these books.

	Kcal	Pro	Cho	Fat	Sfa	Dfib
BEVERAGES						
Alcoholic						
Beer, 12 fl oz	146	0.9	13.2	0	0	0
Beer, light, 12 fl oz	100	0.7	4.8	0	0	0
Wine, table, red, 3.5 fl oz	74	0.2	1.8	0	0	0
Wine, table, white, 3.5 fl oz	70	0.1	0.8	0	0	0
Distilled spirits, 90 proof, 1.5 fl oz	116	0	0	0	0	0
Carbonated Beverages						
Cola, 12 fl oz	151	0.1	38.5	0.1	0	0
Lemon-lime soda, 12 fl oz	141	0	38.4	0	0	0
Tonic/quinine water, 12 fl oz	125	0	32.3	0	0	0
Carbonated Beverages, Low Calorie						
Club soda, 12 fl oz	0	0	0	0	0	0
Diet cola, 12 fl oz	0	0	0	0	0	0
Fruit Juices and Flavored Drinks						
Orange juice, frozen concentrate, 6 fl oz	91	0	22.7	0	0	0
Coffee, brewed, 6 fl oz	4	0.1	0.8	0	0	0
Tea, hot/iced, brewed 3 minutes, 6 fl oz	2	0	0	0.4	0	0

Source: From Jean A.T. Pennington, *Food Values of Portions Commonly Used*, 15th ed. Copyright © 1989 by Jean A.T. Pennington; copyright © 1985, 1980 by Helen Nicholls Church and Jean A.T. Pennington. Reprinted by permission of Harper & Row, Publishers, Inc.

	Kcal	Pro	Cho	Fat	Sfa	Dfib
BEVERAGES (*cont.*)						
Water						
Municipal, 8 fl oz	0	0	0	0	0	0
CEREALS						
Cooked or to Be Cooked						
Cream of rice, cooked, ¾ cup	95	1.6	21.1	0.1		
Cream of wheat, cooked, ¾ cup	115	3.3	23.8	0.4		
Oatmeal, instant, 1 packet prepared	104	4.4	18.1	1.0		
Ready-to-Eat						
Almond Delight, ¾ cup	110	2.1	23	1.6		1.5
Bran, ⅓ cup	71	4	21.1	0.5		8.5
Bran Buds, ⅓ cup	73	3.9	21.6	0.7		7.9
Bran Chex, ⅔ cup	90	2.9	23	0.7		6.1
Bran Flakes						
Kellogg's, ¾ cup	93	3.6	22.2	0.5		4
Post, ⅔ cup	87	3	22.2	0.4	0.1	5.6
Ralston Purina, ⅔ cup	92	3.3	22.6	0.4	0.1	3.5
Cheerios, 1¼ cup	111	4.3	19.6	1.8	0.3	2
Corn Chex, 1 cup	110	2	25	0.2		1.1
Corn Flakes						
Country, General Mills, 1 cup	110	2	25	1		1.1
Kellogg's, 1¼ cup	110	2.3	24.4	0.1		0.3
Ralston Purina, 1 cup	110	2	25	0.1		1.4
Cracklin Bran, ⅓ cup	110	2.6	19.4	4.1		4.3

	Kcal	Pro	Cho	Fat	Sfa	Dfib
CEREALS (*cont.*)						
C.W. Post, ¼ cup	126	2.6	20.3	4.4	3.3	0.7
Fiber One, ½ cup	60	4	21	1		12
Frosted Mini-Wheats, 4 bisquits	102	2.9	23.4	0.3		2.1
Fruit and Fiber, Harvest Medley, ½ cup	91	2.8	21.7	1	0.1	4.2
Golden Grahams, ¾ cup	109	1.6	24.1	1.1	0.8	0.5
Granola						
Hearty, Post, ¼ cup	127	2.4	20.7	4.1	3	0.9
Post, ¼ cup	123	2.2	20.8	3.8	2.7	0.9
Grape-Nut Flakes, ⅞ cup	104	2.8	22.7	0.8	0.4	1.9
Grape-Nuts, ¼ cup	104	3.1	23.1	0.1	0	1.8
Heartland Natural, ¼ cup	123	2.9	19.4	4.4		1.3
Honey Nut Cheerios, ¾ cup	107	3.1	22.8	0.7	0.1	
Kix, 1½ cup	110	2.5	23.4	0.7	0.2	0.4
Life, ⅔ cup	111	5.2	18.6	1.8		0.9
Most, ⅔ cup	95	4	21.6	0.3		3.5
Nutrigrain						
barley, ¾ cup	106	3.1	23.5	0.2		1.7
corn, ⅔ cup	108	2.3	23.9	0.7		1.8
wheat, ¾ cup	102	2.5	24	0.3		1.8
Puffed Rice, 1 cup	57	0.9	12.8	0.1		0.1
100% Natural, ¼ cup	136	3.7	17.8	5.6		1
Raisin Bran						
Kellogg's, ¾ cup	115	4	27.9	0.7		4
Post, ½ cup	86	2.2	22	0.4	0	3.7
Ralston Purina, ¾ cup	120	3	31.4	0.2		4.8
Rice Chex, 1⅛ cup	110	1.7	25	0.3		0.5

	Kcal	Pro	Cho	Fat	Sfa	Dfib
CEREALS (*cont.*)						
Rice Krispies, 1 cup	112	1.9	24.8	0.2		0.1
Shredded Wheat, 1 biscuit	83	2.6	18.8	0.3		2.2
Special K, 1$\frac{1}{3}$ cup	111	5.6	21.3	0.1		0.2
Team, 1 cup	111	1.8	24.3	0.5		0.3
Total, 1 cup	100	2.8	22.3	0.6	0.1	2
Trix, 1 cup	109	1.5	25.2	0.4		0.1
Wheat Chex, $\frac{2}{3}$ cup	100	2.9	23	0.7		3.7
Wheaties, 1 cup	99	2.7	22.6	0.5	0.1	2
CHEESE AND CHEESE PRODUCTS						
American, 1 oz	106	6.3	0.5	8.9	5.6	0
Blue, 1 oz	100	6.1	0.7	8.2	5.3	0
Brick, 1 oz	105	6.6	0.8	8.4	5.3	0
Camembert, 1 oz	85	5.6	0.1	6.9	4.3	0
Caraway, 1 oz	107	7.1	0.9	8.3		0
Cheddar, 1 oz	114	7.1	0.4	9.4	6	0
Cheddar, grated, 1 cup	455	28.1	1.5	37.5	23.8	0
Colby, 1 oz	112	6.7	0.7	9.1	5.7	0
Cottage cheese, creamed, 1 cup	217	26.2	5.6	9.5	6	0
Cottage cheese, low fat, 1% fat, 1 cup	164	28	6.2	2.3	1.5	0
Cottage cheese, low fat, 2% fat, 1 cup	203	31.1	8.2	4.4	2.8	0
Cream cheese, 1 oz	99	2.1	0.8	9.9	6.2	0
Cream cheese, light, Philadelphia, 1 oz	62	2.9	1.8	4.7	2.8	0
Edam, 1 oz	101	7.1	0.4	7.9	5	0
Feta, 1 oz	75	4	1.2	6	4.2	0
Gouda, 1 oz	101	7.1	0.6	7.8	5	0
Gruyere, 1 oz	117	8.5	0.1	9.2	5.4	0

	Kcal	Pro	Cho	Fat	Sfa	Dfib
CHEESE AND CHEESE PRODUCTS (*cont.*)						
Harvarti, 1 oz	121	6.1	0.3	10.6	6.5	0
Limburger, 1 oz	93	5.7	0.1	7.7	4.8	0
Monterey, 1 oz	106	6.9	0.2	8.6		0
Mozzarella, 1 oz	80	5.5	0.6	6.1	3.7	0
Mozzarella, low moisture, 1 oz	90	6.1	0.7	7	4.4	0
Mozzarella, part skim, 1 oz	72	6.9	0.8	4.5	2.9	0
Muenster, 1 oz	104	6.6	0.3	8.5	5.4	0
Neufchatel, 1 oz	74	2.8	0.8	6.6	4.2	0
Parmesan, grated, 1 tablespoon	23	2.1	0.2	1.5	1	0
Pimento, processed, 1 oz	106	6.3	0.5	8.8	5.6	0
Provolone, 1 oz	100	7.3	0.6	7.6	4.8	0
Ricotta, ½ cup	216	14	3.8	16.1	10.3	0
Romano, 1 oz	110	9	1	7.6		0
Swiss, 1 oz	107	8.1	7.8	5		0
American cheese food, 1 oz	93	5.6	2.1	7	4.4	0
Cheese spreads						
American, 1 tablespoon	47	2.7	1.4	3.4	2.2	0
American, 1 oz	82	4.7	2.5	6	3.8	0
Cheese Whiz, 1 oz	77	4.6	1.8	5.7	3.1	0
Velveeta, 1 oz	84	5.2	2.2	6.1	3.6	0
CHIPS, POPCORN, PRETZELS, AND SIMILAR SNACK FOODS						
Popcorn, popped, 1 cup	23	0.8	4.6	0.3	0	
fat and salt added, 1 cup	41	0.9	5.3	2	0.9	
microwave, frozen, butter flavor, 3 cups	192	2.8	18.9	11.5		

	Kcal	Pro	Cho	Fat	Sfa	Dfib
CHIPS, POPCORN, PRETZELS, AND SIMILAR SNACK FOODS (*cont.*)						
original flavor, 3 cups	192	2.8	18.9	11.5		
Potato chips, 1 oz	148	1.8	14.7	10.1	2.6	
Pringles, 1 oz	167	1.6	10.8	13		
Light Style, 1 oz	147	1.9	16.5	8.2		
Pretzels, 1 oz	111	2.6	22.4	1		
Tortilla chips, 1 oz	150	2	18	8		
CREAMS AND CREAM SUBSTITUTES						
Creamers						
liquid, coffee rich, nondairy, ½ fl oz	22	0	2.1	1.6	0.3	0
powdered, 1 teaspoon	11	0.1	1.1	0.7	0.7	0
half-and-half, 1 tablespoon	20	0.4	0.6	1.7	1.1	0
Sour cream, cultured, 1 tablespoon	26	0.4	0.5	2.5	1.6	0
Whipping cream, heavy, 1 tablespoon	52	.3	.4	5.6	3.5	0
DESSERTS						
Brownies, from mix, 1 brownie	86	1	12.6	4	0.8	
Cakes						
angel food, cake mix, Duncan Hines, 1/12 package	131	3.4	28.9	0.2		
homemade, 1 piece	161	4.8	35.7	0.1		
carrot mix, Duncan Hines, 1/12 package	187	1.6	36.1	4		
cheesecake from mix, Jello, ⅛ cheesecake	278	4.9	36.3	12.9	8	

	Kcal	Pro	Cho	Fat	Sfa	Dfib
DESSERTS (*cont.*)						
devil's food, with chocolate icing, homemade, 1 piece	233	2.6	34.2	10.8		
German chocolate, from mix, Pillsbury, $\frac{1}{12}$ cake	250	3	36	11		
pound, from mix, Dromedary, $\frac{1}{2}''$ slice	150	2	21	6		
sponge, 1 piece	188	4.8	35.7	3.1		
white, with chocolate icing, homemade, 1 piece	298	3.3	45.8	12.1		
yellow, with chocolate icing, homemade, 1 piece	292	3.2	43.8	12.3		
Cookies (commercial unless otherwise indicated)						
Animal Crackers, 10 pieces	112	1.7	20.8	2.4	0.6	
Apple Newtons, 2 cookies	147	1.3	28	2.7		
chocolate chip, 2 cookies	99	1.1	14.6	4.4		
chocolate sandwich, 1 cookie	49	0.5	7.1	2.1		
Fig Newtons, 2 cookies	100	1	20	2		
peanut butter, Almost Home, 2 cookies	140	3	16	7		
refrigerated dough, 1 cookie	50	0.8	5.9	2.6		

	Kcal	Pro	Cho	Fat	Sfa	Dfib
DESSERTS (*cont.*)						
sugar, homemade, 2 cookies	71	1	10.9	2.7	0.7	
vanilla wafers, 5 cookies	92	1.1	14.9	3.2		
Doughnuts						
cake, 1 doughnut	105	1.3	12.2	5.8		
yeast, 1 doughnut	176	2.7	16	11.3	2.8	
Frozen desserts						
frozen yogurt, Honey Hill Farms, 4.5 fl oz	118	3.5	18.7	3.5		
fruit juice bar, Jello, 1 bar	42	0.6	10.1	0	0	0
ice cream, vanilla, Haagen-Dazs, ½ cup	270	5	24	17	11.0	0
ice milk, vanilla, 1 cup	184	5.2	29	5.6	3.5	0
sherbet, orange, 1 cup	270	2.2	58.7	2.4		0
sorbet, peach, Dole, ½ cup	120	0.6	29.6	0.1		0
Gelatin, all flavors						
Jello, ½ cup	81	1.6	18.8	0	0	0
Sugar free, D-Zerta, ½ cup	8	1.6	0.1	0	0	0
Pastries						
Danish, 1 pastry	161	2.6	18.8	8.8		0
eclair, chocolate, 1 eclair	205	2.3	27.3	9.7		0
sweet roll, cinnamon, 1 roll	154	2.6	21.4	6.8		0

	Kcal	Pro	Cho	Fat	Sfa	Dfib
DESSERTS (*cont.*)						
Pies						
apple, frozen, baked, ⅛ pie	231	1.8	36.5	9.1	2.3	
cherry, ⅛ pie	308	4.1	45.3	13.3	3.5	
pecan, ⅛ pie	430	5.3	52.8	23.6	3.3	
pumpkin, ⅛ pie	241	4.6	27.9	12.8	4.5	
strawberry, ⅛ pie	184	1.8	28.7	7.3	1.8	
Puddings						
all flavors, instant mix, Royal, ½ cup	181	3.7	31.5	4.4		0
instant mix, sugar free, Royal, ½ cup	103	4.3	16.3	2.3		0
Sauces, Syrups, and Toppings for Desserts						
Chocolate syrup, 2 tablespoons	92	0.9	23.5	0.8	0.4	0
fudge topping, 2 tablespoons	124	1.9	20.3	5.1	2.9	0
icing/frosting, ready to spread, all flavors, General Mills, $\frac{1}{12}$ tube	164	1	23.9	7.3		0
EGGS, EGG DISHES, AND EGG SUBSTITUTES						
Boiled, 1 large egg	79	6.1	0.6	5.6	1.7	0
Fried, 1 large egg	83	5.4	0.5	6.4	2.4	0
Poached, 1 large egg	70	6	0.6	5.6	1.7	0
Scrambled with milk and fat, 1 large egg	95	6	1.4	7.1	0.7	0
White, 1 large egg	16	3.4	0.4	0	0	0
Yolk, 1 large egg	63	2.8	0	5.6	1.7	0

	Kcal	Pro	Cho	Fat	Sfa	Dfib
EGGS, EGG DISHES, AND EGG SUBSTITUTES (*cont.*)						
Omelette, cheddar cheese, frozen, Am Hospital Company, 4 oz	313	15.9	1.3	27.1		0
Quiche, bacon and onion, Pour a Quiche, 4.3 oz	230	13.0	6	18		
Egg substitute, frozen, ¼ cup	96	6.8	1.9	6.7	1.2	0
ENTREES AND MEALS						
Box Mix Entrees						
Chicken Helper, ⅕ package with chicken	530	32.6	36.8	27.8		0
Hamburger Helper, ⅕ package with ⅕ ground beef	335	19.4	33.8	14.9		0
macaroni and cheese, Kraft deluxe dinner, ¾ cup	225	10.8	36.3	7.5	4.2	0
Tuna Helper, ⅕ package with 1.3 oz tuna	300	14.8	29	13.8		0
Canned Entrees						
beans, baked, with beef, 1 cup	321	17	45	9.2	4.5	
beef ravioli, Franco-American, 7.5 oz	233	9	36.1	4.7		
chicken and vegetable stew, Bounty, 7.5 oz	166	10.5	15.1	7		

	Kcal	Pro	Cho	Fat	Sfa	Dfib
ENTREES AND MEALS (*cont.*)						
chili with beans, 1 cup	286	14.6	30.4	14	6	
linguine with white clam sauce, Prego, 11 oz	391	17.8	56.4	10.5		
macaroni and cheese, 1 cup	228	9.4	25.7	9.6	4.2	
noodles and chicken, Bounty, 7.5 oz	204	17.9	16.8	11.7		
ravioli with meat sauce, Franco-American, 7.5 oz	284	11.3	35.4	10.8		
spaghetti with meat sauce, Franco-American, 7.5 oz	211	8.5	26.2	8.1		
spaghetti with tomato sauce, Franco-American, 7.4 oz	171	5.1	35	1.2		
Frozen Entrees						
beef burgundy, Light and Elegant, 9 oz entree	230	23	25	4		
beef sliced, and vegetable, Banquet, 10 oz entree	300	38	17	9		
beef stew, Banquet, ¼ of 32 oz package	254	12	21	13		
beef stroganoff, Light and Elegant, 9 oz entree	260	24	27	6		
burrito, beef, El Charrito, 5 oz burrito	340	10	39	17		

	Kcal	Pro	Cho	Fat	Sfa	Dfib
ENTREES AND MEALS (*cont.*)						
chicken a la king, Banquet, 4 oz entree	110	8	9	5		
chicken and dumplings, ¼ of 32 oz package	430	18	31	25		
chicken, glazed, with vegetable rice, Light and Elegant, 8 oz entree	240	29	23	4		
chicken parmigiana, Light and Elegant, 8 oz entree	260	28	23	6		
chicken with broccoli, Light and Elegant, 9.5 oz entree	290	19	30	11		
enchiladas						
beef and cheese, El Charrito, 6 enchiladas	880	23	96	42		
cheese, El Charrito, 3 enchiladas	470	12	64	20		
chicken, El Charrito, 3 enchiladas	440	23	59	13		
fish, batter dipped, and chips						
Van de Kamp's, 7 oz entree	440	20	35	25		
florentine, Light and Elegant, 11.25 oz entree	280	24	35	5		

	Kcal	Pro	Cho	Fat	Sfa	Dfib
ENTREES AND MEALS (*cont.*)						
green pepper steak, Banquet, 10 oz entree	310	21	44	5		
macaroni and cheese						
Banquet, 8 oz entree	344	11	36	17		
Light and Elegant, 9 oz entree	300	16	38	9		
meatloaf, Banquet, 5 oz entree	240	12	12	15		
pizza, cheese						
Pillsbury Microwave, 7.1 oz	480	21	56	19		
pizza combination						
Pillsbury Microwave, 9 oz	673	29.7	59.4	36.2		
pizza, pepperoni						
Pillsbury Microwave, 8.5 oz	595	26.8	59.5	28		
Totino's Classic, ¼ pizza	409	17.2	40.3	19.9		
pizza, sausage						
Pillsbury Microwave, 8.75 oz	647	25.3	59	34.2		
Totino's Classic, ¼ pizza	439	16.2	40.5	23.5		
pizza, sausage and pepperoni						
Pillsbury Microwave, Heat and Eat, 4.9 oz	378	13.9	31.3	21.3		

	Kcal	Pro	Cho	Fat	Sfa	Dfib
ENTREES AND MEALS (*cont.*)						
Totino's Party, ⅓ pizza	278	10.5	30.9	15.5		
pizza, vegetable						
Totino's Party, ⅓ pizza	219	7.9	29.2	7.9		
salisbury steak, Banquet, 5 oz entree	230	10	7	18		
scrod fillet						
with broccoli and mozzarella, Seafood Elites, 5 oz entree	140	19	1	7		
with lemon and wild rice, Seafood Elites, 5 oz entree	150	20	7	5		
shrimp creole, Light and Elegant, 10 oz entree	218	14	36	2		
sirloin tips, Banquet, 10 oz entree	160	13	24	1		
sole fillet						
with broccoli and mozzarella, Seafood Elites, 5 oz entree	150	18	2	7		
with lemon and wild rice, Seafood Elites, 5 oz entree	150	16	8	7		
spaghetti with meat sauce						
Banquet, 8 oz entree	270	14	35	8		

	Kcal	Pro	Cho	Fat	Sfa	Dfib
ENTREES AND MEALS (*cont.*)						
Light and Elegant, 10.25 oz entree	290	16	40	8		
sweet and sour pork Van de Kamp's, 11 oz entree	430	15	65	15		
tostada, beef supreme, Van de Kamp's, 8.5 oz entree	530	25	40	30		
turkey, sliced with gravy, Banquet, 5 oz entree	110	8.6	7	5		
veal parmigiana, Banquet, 5 oz entree	230	10	20	11		
Frozen Meals (Usually 3-Course Meals)						
Beef						
Banquet, Extra Helping, 10 oz meal	864	40	72	46		
beef burgundy, Armour Dinner Classics, 10.5 oz meal	330	28	23	15		
beef stroganoff, Armour Dinner Classics, 11.25 oz meal	370	25	21	21		
Chicken						
chicken a la king, Le Menu, 10.25 oz meal	320	22	29	13		
chicken and dumplings, Banquet, 9 oz meal	286	13	28	13		

	Kcal	Pro	Cho	Fat	Sfa	Dfib
ENTREES AND MEALS (*cont.*)						
chicken breasts medallions, Armour Classic Lites, 11 oz meal	20	22	28	7		
fried, Banquet, 11 oz meal	359	18	46	11		
oriental, Armour Classic Lites, 10 oz meal	250	24	26	6		
roasted, Armour Classic Lites, 10 oz meal	250	24	26	6		
chopped sirloin, Le Menu, 12.25 oz meal	410	26	28	23		
cod, almandine, Armour Dinner Classics, 12 oz meal	360	23	33	15		
Enchilada						
beef and cheese, Van de Kamp's, 14.75 oz meal	540	25	60	20		
beef, Banquet, 12 oz meal	497	19	15	72		
cheese, Banquet, 12 oz meal	542	22	71	19		
chicken, Van de Kamp's, 14.75 oz meal	550	25	20	65		
Fillet of fish, Van de Kamp's, 12 oz meal	300	25	25	10		

	Kcal	Pro	Cho	Fat	Sfa	Dfib
ENTREES AND MEALS (*cont.*)						
Fish, Banquet, 8.75 oz meal	553	18	45	33		
Ham, Banquet, 10 oz meal	532	21	61	22		
Imperial chicken, Weight Watchers, 9.25 oz meal	240	22	29	4		
Lasagna, Armour Dinner Classics, 10 oz meal	380	17	42	16		
Macaroni and cheese, Banquet, 9 oz meal	334	11	37	16		
Meat loaf, Banquet, 11 oz meal	437	20	30	27		
Noodles and chicken, Banquet, 9.5 oz meal	361	13	50	11		
Oriental beef, Lean Cuisine, 8.6 oz meal	270	20	30	8		
Salisbury steak						
Banquet, 11 oz meal	395	17	24	26		
Italian style, Lean Cuisine, 9.5 oz meal	270	25	14	13		
with broccoli, Armour Classic Lites, 10 oz meal	290	20	25	13		
with potatoes, Armour Dinner Classics, 11 oz meal	480	20	39	27		
Shrimp, Armour Dinner Classics, 11.5 oz meal	280	18	31	10		

	Kcal	Pro	Cho	Fat	Sfa	Dfib
ENTREES AND MEALS (*cont.*)						
Shrimp in cream sauce, Armour Classic Lites, 10.5 oz meal	280	17	34	8		
Sirloin tips, Armour Dinner Classics, 11 oz meal	370	290	27	16		
Spaghetti and meatballs						
Armour Dinner Classics, 11 oz meal	350	14	27	21		
Banquet, 9.5 oz meal	418	15	57	14		
Stuffed cabbage, Armour Classic Lites, 12 oz meal	290	13	43	8		
Stuffed green peppers, Armour Dinner Classics, 12 oz meal	390	16	41	18		
Swedish meatballs, Armour Dinner Classics, 11.5 oz meal	470	23	32	28		
Sweet and sour chicken						
Armour Classic Lites, 11 oz meal	250	23	33	3		
Armour Dinner Classics, 11 oz meal	450	16	51	20		
Szechuan beef, Armour Classic Lites, 10 oz meal	280	23	26	9		
Teriyaki chicken, Armour Dinner Classics, 10.5 oz meal	250	28	22	5		

	Kcal	Pro	Cho	Fat	Sfa	Dfib
ENTREES AND MEALS (*cont.*)						
Teriyaki steak, Armour Dinner Classics, 10 oz meal	360	24	32	16		
Turf and surf, Armour Classic Lites, 10 oz meal	250	31	14	7		
Turkey, Banquet, 11 oz meal	320	19	41	9		
Veal parmigiana, Banquet, 11 oz meal	413	14	43	21		
Homemade Entrees						
Beef and vegetable stew, 1 cup	218	15.7	15.2	10.5	4.9	
Chicken and noodles, 1 cup	367	22.3	25.7	18.5	5.9	
Chop suey, 1 cup	300	26	12.8	17	8.5	
Crab, deviled, 1 cup	451	27.4	31.9	22.6		
Fish cake, fried, 1 piece	103	8.8	5.6	4.8		
Green pepper, stuffed, 1 pepper	315	24.1	31.1	10.2	4.8	
Macaroni and cheese, 1 cup	430	16.8	40.2	22.2	11	
Salmon patty, 3.5 oz	239	15.8	16.1	12.4		
Salmon rice loaf, 1 slice	212	20.9	12.7	7.8		
Spaghetti in tomato sauce, 1 cup	260	8.8	37	8.8		
Spaghetti with meatballs, 1 cup	332	18.6	38.7	8.8	2	
Tuna patty, 3.5 oz	209	19.8	7.4	0.7		

	Kcal	Pro	Cho	Fat	Sfa	Dfib
FATS, OILS, AND SHORTENINGS						
Animal Fat						
Beef suet, 1 oz	242	0.4	0	26.7	14.8	
Chicken fat, 1 tablespoon	115	0	0	12.8	3.8	
Pork fat (lard), 1 tablespoon	115	0	0	12.8	5	
Turkey fat, 1 tablespoon	115	0	0	12.8	3.8	
Vegetable Oils						
Coconut oil, 1 tablespoon	120	0	0	13.6	11.8	
Corn oil, 1 tablespoon	120	0	0	13.6	1.7	
Cottonseed oil, 1 tablespoon	120	0	0	13.6	3.5	
Olive oil, 1 tablespoon	119	0	0	13.5	1.8	
Palm oil, 1 tablespoon	120	0	0	13.6	6.7	
Palm kernel oil, 1 tablespoon	120	0	0	13.6	11.1	
Peanut oil, 1 tablespoon	130	0	0	14	2	
Popcorn oil, Planters, 1 tablespoon	130	0	0	14	0.2	
Safflower oil, 1 tablespoon	120	0	0	13.6	1.2	
Sesame oil, 1 tablespoon	120	0	0	13.6	1.9	
Soybean oil, 1 tablespoon	120	0	0	13.6	2	
Soybean oil, hydrogenated, 1 tablespoon	120	0	0	13.6	2	
Sunflower oil, 1 tablespoon	120	0	0	13.6	1.4	

	Kcal	Pro	Cho	Fat	Sfa	Dfib
FATS, OILS, AND SHORTENINGS (*cont.*)						
Vegetable oil spray						
Mazola No Stick, 2.5-second spray	6	0	0	0.7	0.1	
Shortenings						
Lard and vegetable, 1 tablespoon	115	0	0	12.8	5.2	
FISH, SHELLFISH, AND CRUSTACEANS						
Abalone, fried, 3 oz	161	16.7	9.4	5.8	1.4	0
Anchovy, 3 oz	111	17.3	0	4.1	1.1	0
Anchovy paste, 1 teaspoon	14	1.4	0.3	0.8	0.5	0
Bluefish, 3 oz	105	17	0	3.6	0.8	0
Catfish						
channel, 3 oz	99	15.5	0	3.6	0.8	0
breaded and fried, 3 oz	194	15.4	11.3	6.9	2.8	0
Caviar, 1 tablespoon	40	3.9	0.6	2.9		0
Clams						
raw, 3 oz	63	10.9	2.2	0.8	0.1	0
breaded and fried, 3 oz	171	12.1	8.8	9.5	2.3	0
canned, 3 oz	126	21.7	4.4	1.7	0.2	0
Cod, Atlantic/Pacific, 3 oz	70	15.1	0	0.6	0.1	0
Crab						
Alaska king, 3 oz	71	15.6	0	0.5		0
dungeness, 3 oz	73	14.8	0.6	0.8	0.1	
imitation, 3 oz	87	10.2	8.7	1.1		0
Crab cakes, 1 cake	93	12.1	0.3	4.5	0.9	
Crayfish, 3 oz	76	15.9	0	0.9	0.2	

	Kcal	Pro	Cho	Fat	Sfa	Dfib
FISH, SHELLFISH, AND CRUSTACEANS (*cont.*)						
Fish fillet						
batter dipped, Van de Kamp's, 3-oz piece	180	10	15	10		
light and crispy, Van de Kamp's, 2-oz piece	180	5	10	15		
Fish kabobs, Van de Kamp's, 4 oz	240	10	15	15		
Fish sticks						
frozen, batter dipped, Van de Kamp's, 4 pieces	220	10	15	15		
light and crispy, Van de Kamp's, 4 pieces	270	10	15	20		
Flounder/sole, 3 oz	68	14.9	0	0.5		0
Flounder/sole						
baked, 3.5 oz	202	30	0	8.2		0
frozen, breaded, Van de Kamp's, 5-oz piece	300	15	15	15		0
Grouper, 3 oz	78	16.5	0	0.9	0.2	0
Haddock, 3 oz	74	16.1	0	0.6	0.1	0
frozen, batter dipped, Van de Kamp's, 2 pieces	240	10	20	10		0
frozen, breaded, Van de Kamp's, 5-oz piece	300	15	15	20		0
frozen, light and crispy, Van de Kamp's, 2-oz piece	180	5	10	15		0

	Kcal	Pro	Cho	Fat	Sfa	Dfib
FISH, SHELLFISH, AND CRUSTACEANS (*cont.*)						
smoked, 3 oz	99	21.4	0	0.8	0.1	0
Halibut, Atlantic and Pacific, 3 oz	93	17.7	0	2	0.3	0
Halibut, frozen						
batter-dipped, Van de Kamp's, 3-oz piece	260	10	15	15		0
breaded, Van de Kamp's, 4-oz piece	220	15	15	10		
Herring, Atlantic, 3 oz	134	15.3	0	7.7	1.7	0
Herring, Atlantic, pickled, 1 piece	39	2.1	1.5	2.7	0.4	
Lobster, 3 oz	77	16	0.4	0.8		
paste, 1 teaspoon	13	1.5	0.1	0.7		0
salad, 3.5 oz	110	10.1	2.3	6.4		
Mackerel, king, 3 oz	89	17.2	0	1.7	0.3	0
Ocean perch, 3 oz	80	15.8	0	1.4	0.2	0
Oysters, 6 med.	58	5.9	3.3	2.1	0.5	0
breaded and fried, 3 oz	167	7.5	9.9	10.7	2.7	0
canned, 3 oz	117	12	6.7	4.2	1.1	0
Perch, 3 oz	77	16.5	0	0.8	0.2	0
Perch, frozen, batter-dipped, Van de Kamp's, 2 pieces	270	10	20	15		0
Perch, fillet, light and crispy, Van de Kamp's, 3 oz	170	5	10	10		0
Pompano, 3 oz	40	15.7	0	8.1	3	0
Roughy, orange, 3 oz	107	12.5	0	6	0.1	0
Salmon						
Atlantic, 3 oz	121	16.9	0	5.4	0.8	0

	Kcal	Pro	Cho	Fat	Sfa	Dfib
FISH, SHELLFISH, AND CRUSTACEANS (*cont.*)						
chinook, 3 oz	153	17.1	0	8.9	2.1	0
chinook, smoked, 3 oz	99	15.5	0	8.9	2.1	0
chum, 3 oz	102	17.1	0	3.2	0.7	0
canned with bone, 3 oz	120	18.2	0	4.7	1.3	
pink, 3 oz	99	17	0	2.9	0.5	0
sockeye, 3 oz	143	18.1	0	7.3	1.6	0
canned with bone, 3 oz	130	17.4	0	6.2	1.4	
Sardines						
Atlantic, canned in soybean oil, 2 sardines	50	5.9	0	2.8	0.4	
Pacific, canned in tomato sauce, 1 sardine	68	6.2	0	4.6	1.2	
Scallops						
breaded and fried, 3 oz	75	14.3	2	0.6	0.1	0
2 large	67	5.6	3.1	3.4	0.8	
Shrimp						
3 oz (12 large)	90	17.8	0.8	1.5	0.3	
breaded and fried, 3 oz (11 large)	206	18.2	9.8	10.4	1.8	
canned, 3 oz	102	19.6	0.9	1.7	0.3	
french fried, 3.5 oz	225	20.3	10	10.8		
frozen, breaded, 3.5 oz	139	12.3	19.9	0.7		
imitation, 3 oz	86	10.5	7.8	1.3		
Smelt, Atlantic, 4–5 medium	98	18.6	2.1	0		

	Kcal	Pro	Cho	Fat	Sfa	Dfib
FISH, SHELLFISH, AND CRUSTACEANS (*cont.*)						
Snapper, 3 oz	85	17.4	0	1.1	0.2	0
Sole, 3.5 oz	68	14.9	0	0.5		0
batter-dipped, Van de Kamp's, 2 pieces	250	15	25	15		
breaded, Van de Kamp's, 5-oz piece	300	15	15	15		
Swordfish, 3 oz	103	16.8	0	3.4	0.9	
Trout, rainbow, 3 oz	100	17.5	0	2.9	0.6	0
Tuna						
canned in oil, light, 3 oz	169	24.8	0	7	1.3	0
canned in spring water, light, 3 oz	11	25.1	0	0.4	0.1	0
salad, ½ cup	383	32.9	19.3	19	3.2	
yellowfin, 3 oz	92	19.9	0	0.8	0.2	0
Whitefish						
baked, stuffed, 3.5 oz	215	15.2	5.8	14		
smoked, 3 oz	92	19.9	0	0.8	0.2	0
VEGETABLE JUICES AND FRUITS						
Vegetable Juices						
Carrot juice, canned, 8 fl oz	73	1.7	17.1	0.3	0.1	
Clam and tomato juice, canned, 5.5 fl oz	77	1.1	19.1	0.1	0	
Cranberry juice cocktail, bottled, 8 fl oz	147	0.1	37.7	0.1		
Grape juice, canned/bottled, 8 fl oz	155	1.4	37.9	0.2	0.1	0

	Kcal	Pro	Cho	Fat	Sfa	Dfib
VEGETABLE JUICES AND FRUITS (*cont.*)						
Grapefruit juice, canned, 8 fl oz	93	1.3	22.1	0.2	0	
Lemon juice, fresh, 1 tablespoon	4	0.1	1.3	0		
Orange juice, canned, 8 fl oz	104	1.5	24.5	0.4	0	
Orange juice, frozen concentrate, 8 fl oz	112	1.7	26.8	0.1	0	
Tomato juice, 6 fl oz	32	1.4	7.7	0.4	0	
Tomato juice cocktail, canned, 8 fl oz	51	1.7	12.2	0.2		
Vegetable juice cocktail, canned, 6 fl oz	34	1.1	8.3	0.2	0	
V-8 vegetable cocktail, Campbell's, 6 fl oz	37	1.3	7.8	0		
spicy hot, 6 fl oz	37	1.5	7.8	0		
Fruits						
Apple						
raw, with skin, 1 medium	81	0.3	21.1	0.5	0.1	2.8
raw, without skin, 1 medium	72	0.2	19	0.4	0.1	2.9
canned, sliced, sweetened, ½ cup	68	0.2	17	0.5	0.1	1.9
Applesauce						
canned, sweetened, ½ cup	97	0.2	25.5	0.2	0	1.4
canned, unsweetened, ½ cup	53	0.2	13.8	0.1		1.4
Apricots, 3 medium	51	1.5	11.8	0.4	0	1.4

	Kcal	Pro	Cho	Fat	Sfa	Dfib
VEGETABLE JUICES AND FRUITS (*cont.*)						
canned, heavy syrup, 4 halves	75	0.5	19.3	0.1	0	
canned, juice packed, 4 halves	40	0.5	10.4	0	0	0.4
canned, light syrup, 3 halves	54	0.5	14	0	0	
Banana, 1 medium	105	1.2	26.7	0.6	0.2	1.6
Blueberries, 1 cup	82	1	20.5	0.6		4.4
canned, heavy syrup, ½ cup	112	0.8	28.2	0.4		
frozen, sweetened, 1 cup	187	0.9	50.5	.3		
Cantaloupe, 1 cup pieces	57	1.4	13.4	0.4		0.5
Cherries						
sour, canned, heavy syrup, ½ cup	116	0.9	29.8	0.1	0	
sour, canned, water packed, ½ cup	43	0.9	10.9	0.1	0	
sweet, 10 cherries	49	0.8	11.3	0.7	0.1	0
sweet, canned in heavy syrup, ½ cup	107	0.8	27.4	0.2	0	
sweet, canned juice pack, ½ cup	68	1.1	17.3	0	0	0.3
Dates, dried, 10 dates	228	1.6	61	0.4		4.2
Grapefruit						
pink and red, ½ medium	37	0.7	9.5	0.1	0	
canned, juice pack, ½ cup	46	0.9	11.4	0.1	0	
Grapes						
American, 1 cup	58	0.6	15.8	0.3	0.1	

	Kcal	Pro	Cho	Fat	Sfa	Dfib
VEGETABLE JUICES AND FRUITS (*cont.*)						
European, 1 cup	114	1.1	28.4	0.9	0.3	2.6
Thompson, seedless, canned, ½ cup	94	0.6	25.2	0.1	0	
Honeydew melon, ¼ cup	33	0.8	7.7	0.3		
Kiwi fruit, 1 medium	46	0.8	11.3	0.3		
Lemon, 1 medium	17	0.6	5.4	0.2	0	
Lime, 1 medium	20	0.5	7.1	0.1	0	
Mandarin oranges, canned						
juice packed, ½ cup	46	0.8	11.9	0	0	
light syrup, ½ cup	76	.6	20.4	0.1	0	
Mixed fruit						
canned, heavy syrup, ½ cup	92	0.5	24	0.1	0	
dried, 3.5 oz	243	2.5	64.1	0.5	0	
frozen in syrup, Birds Eye, ½ cup	123	0.8	31	0.4	0.1	
frozen, sweetened, 1 cup	245	3.5	60.6	0.5	0.1	
Nectarine, 1 medium	67	1.3	16	0.6		
Orange						
navel, 1 medium	65	1.4	16.3	0.1	0	
Valencia, 1 medium	59	1.3	14.4	0.4	0	
Peach, 1 medium	37	0.6	9.7	0		
canned, heavy syrup, 1 cup	190	1.2	51	0.3	0	
canned, juice packed, 1 cup	109	1.6	28.7	0.1	0	1.1
canned, light syrup, 1 cup	136	1.1	36.5	0.1	0	
canned, water packed, 1 cup	58	1.1	14.9	0.1	0	

	Kcal	Pro	Cho	Fat	Sfa	Dfib
VEGETABLE JUICES AND FRUITS (*cont.*)						
frozen, sweetened, 1 cup	235	1.6	59.0	0.3	0	
Pear, 1 medium	98	0.7	25.1	0.7	0	4.1
canned, heavy syrup, 1 cup	188	0.5	48.9	0.3	0.1	
canned, juice pack, 1 cup	123	0.9	32.1	0.2	0	2.3
canned, light syrup, 1 cup	144	0.5	38.1	0.1	0	
canned, water pack, 1 cup	71	0.5	19.1	0.1	0	
dried, sulfured, 10 halves	459	3.3	122	1.1	0.1	
Pineapple, 1 cup pieces	77	0.6	19.2	0.7	0	2.4
canned, heavy syrup, 1 cup pieces	199	0.9	51.5	0.3	0	
canned, juice pack, 1 cup pieces	150	1	39.2	0.2	0	1.0
Plum, 1 medium	36	0.5	8.6	0.4	0	
heavy syrup, 3 plums	110	0.5	30.9	0.1	0	
canned, juice pack, 3 plums	55	0.5	14.4	0	0	0.4
Prunes, canned, heavy syrup, 5 prunes	90	0.8	23.9	0.2	0	
Raisins						
golden seedless, ⅔ cup	302	3.4	79.5	0.5	0.2	
seedless, ⅔ cup	300	3.2	79.1	0.5	0.2	
Raspberries, 1 cup	61	1.1	14.2	0.7	0	5.8
canned, heavy syrup, ½ cup	117	1.1	29.9	0.2	0	
frozen, in light syrup, Birds Eye, ½ cup	99	0.8	24.6	0.5	0	4.3

	Kcal	Pro	Cho	Fat	Sfa	Dfib
VEGETABLE JUICES AND FRUITS (*cont.*)						
frozen, sweetened, 2/5 cup	103	0.7	26.2	0.2	0	
Strawberries, 1 cup	45	0.9	10.5	0.6	0	2.8
frozen, in light syrup, Birds Eye, 1/2 cup	87	0.7	21.6	0.4	0.2	2.2
frozen, sweetened, 1 cup	245	1.4	66.1	0.3	0.2	
frozen, unsweetened, 1 cup	52	0.6	13.6	0.2	0	
Tangerine, 1 medium	37	0.5	9.4	0.2	0	
Watermelon, 1 cup	50	1	11.5	0.7		0.3
GRAIN FRACTIONS						
Bisquick, General Mills, 2 oz	240	4	37	8		
Oat bran, 1/3 cup	110	5.7	16.2	2.5		
Wheat bran, unprocessed, Quaker, 2 tablespoons	21	1.1	3.6	0.2		
Wheat flour, all-purpose, 1 cup	499	14.4	104.3	1.4		
self-rising, 1 cup	440	11.6	92.8	1.3		
whole wheat, 1 cup	400	16	85.2	1.2		
wheat germ, toasted, 1/4 cup	108	8.3	14.1	3	0.5	3
GRAIN PRODUCTS						
Biscuits						
From mix, 1 biscuit	93	2.1	13.6	3.3		

	Kcal	Pro	Cho	Fat	Sfa	Dfib
GRAIN PRODUCTS (*cont.*)						
From refrigerated dough, 1 biscuit	91	2	13.6	3.1		
Homemade, 1 biscuit	103	2.1	12.8	4.8	1.2	
Baking powder, Pillsbury, 2 biscuits	110	1.9	14	5.3		
Buttermilk, flaky, Hungry Jack, 2 biscuits	171	3.4	24.6	65		
Breads and Bread Products						
Bagel, 1 bagel	163	6	30.9	1.4		
Bread crumbs, dry, 1 cup	392	12.6	73.4	4.6	1.1	
Breadsticks, 2 sticks	77	2.4	15.1	0.6	0.1	
Corn bread, from mix, 1 piece	178	3.8	27.5	5.8	1.7	
French, 1 slice	81	2.7	14.8	1.1		
Wonder, 1 slice	70	3	13	1		
Italian, 1 slice	78	2.8	14.9	0.6		
Mixed grain, 1 slice	64	2.5	11.7	0.9		
Toasted, 1 slice	63	2.4	13	1.2		
Pita pocket, 1 pocket	106	4	20.6	0.6		0.3
Sourdough, 1 slice	70	3	12	1		
Wheat, 1 slice	61	2.3	11.3	1		
toasted, 1 slice	61	2.3	11.3	1		
White, 1 slice	64	2	11.7	0.9		
toasted, 1 slice	64	2	11.7	0.9		
Whole wheat, 1 slice	61	2.4	11.4	1.1		1.6
toasted, 1 slice	59	2.3	10.9	1.1		
Crackers						
Cheese, 5 pieces	81	1.4	7.8	4.9		

	Kcal	Pro	Cho	Fat	Sfa	Dfib
GRAIN PRODUCTS (*cont.*)						
Cheese, Ritz, 5 crackers	70	1	8	3		
Cheese, with peanut butter filling, 6 sandwiches	209	65	23.8	10.2	9	
Graham, 2 crackers	60	1	10	8	1.5	
Nutty wheat thins, Nabisco, 7 crackers	80	1	8	5		
Oyster, 10 crackers	33	0.7	5.3	1	0.2	
Ry-Krisp, ¼ of large square	40	1.5	13	0.2		
Saltines, 2 crackers	26	0.6	4.4	0.6		
Soda, 10 crackers	125	2.6	20.1	3.7	0.9	
Triscuits, 3 crackers	60	1	10	2		
Twigs, sesame, Nabisco, 7 crackers	70	1	8	4		
Waverly, Nabisco, 4 crackers	70	1	10	3		
Wheatsworth, 5 crackers	70	1	9	3		
Wheat Thins, Nabisco, 8 crackers	70	1	9	3		
Zwieback, 1 piece	30	0.7	5.2	0.6	0.2	
French Toast						
Frozen, Aunt Jemima, 2 slices	168	6.4	26.8	3.9		
Raisin, Aunt Jemima, 2 slices	185	7.3	29.4	4.2		
Homemade, 2 slices	153	5.7	17.2	6.7		
Muffins						
Blueberry, from mix, 1 muffin	126	2.4	19.5	4.3		

	Kcal	Pro	Cho	Fat	Sfa	Dfib
GRAIN PRODUCTS (*cont.*)						
Bran, homemade, 1 muffin	112	3	16.7	5.1		
Corn						
from mix, 1 muffin	130	2.8	20	4.2	1.3	
homemade, 1 muffin	126	2.8	19.2	4	1.2	
English						
Plain, 1 muffin	135	4.5	26.2	1.1		
Plain, toasted, 1 muffin	145	4.8	28.1	1.2		
Whole wheat, 1 muffin	130	4	27	1		
Pancakes						
From frozen batter						
buttermilk, Aunt Jemima, 3 4″ pancakes	212	7.1	42.6	1.5		
From mix						
buttermilk, Hungry Jack, 3 4″ pancakes	190	4.2	37.1	2.5		
extra lights, Hungry Jack, 3 4″ pancakes	190	4.2	37.1	2.5		
Homemade						
3 4″ pancakes	186	5.9	27.6	5.9		
Pasta						
Macaroni, 1 cup	159	5.2	3.7	0.7		
Noodles						
chow mein, 1 cup	220	5.9	26.1	10.6		
Muellers, 2 oz dry	220	8	39.8	2.9		
lasagna, Muellers, 2 oz dry	210	7.8	41.6	1.4		

	Kcal	Pro	Cho	Fat	Sfa	Dfib
GRAIN PRODUCTS (*cont.*)						
Spaghetti, 1 cup	159	5.2	33.7	0.7		0.6
Rolls						
Dinner, Home Pride, 1 roll	80	2	14	2		
Dinner pan, 1 roll	85	2.4	12	2.1		
Enriched, 1 roll	137	4.3	28.3	0.4		
Hamburger, 1 roll	114	3.4	20.1	2.1		
Hot dog, 1 roll	114	3.4	20.1	2.1		
Refrigerated dough						
butterflake, 1 roll	110	2.5	16.3	3.8		
crescent, 2 rolls	190	3	25	8		
Sourdough, Earth Grains, 1 roll	100	3	19	1		
Stuffing						
From mix						
bread, 1 cup	416	8.8	39.4	25.6	13.1	
chicken-flavored, Stove Top, ½ cup	176	3.9	20.5	8.8	5	
turkey-flavored, Stove Top, ½ cup	174	3.7	20.6	8.7	5	
wild rice and mushroom, Stove Top, ½ cup	205	3.7	20.6	12.4	7.3	
Tortillas						
Corn, 1 tortilla	67	2.1	12.8	1.1		1
Tostada/taco shell, 1 shell	50	1	7.2	2.2		

	Kcal	Pro	Cho	Fat	Sfa	Dfib
GRAIN PRODUCTS (*cont.*)						
Flour, 2 tortillas	170	5	30	4		
Waffles						
Frozen, buttermilk, Aunt Jemima, 2 waffles	175	4.6	29	4.3		
Plain, Aunt Jemima, 2 waffles	173	4.6	29	4.3		
MEATS						
Beef						
Brisket						
separated lean and fat, braised, 3.5 oz	391	23	0	32.4	13.2	0
separated lean, braised, 3.5 oz	241	29.4	0	12.8	4.6	0
Chuck arm pot roast						
separated lean and fat, braised, 3.5 oz	350	27.1	0	26	10.7	0
separated lean, braised, 3.5 oz	231	33	0	10	3.8	0
Chuck blade roast						
separated lean and fat, braised, 3.5 oz	383	25.4	0	15.3	6.2	0
separated lean, braised, 3.5 oz	270	31.10	15.3	6.2	0	
Corned beef						
cured brisket, 3.5 oz	251	18.2	0.5	19.6.3		
dried, 1 oz	47	8.3	0.4	1.1	0.5	
Flank						
separated lean and fat, braised, 3.5 oz	257	27.5	0	15.5	6.6	0

	Kcal	Pro	Cho	Fat	Sfa	Dfib
MEATS (*cont.*)						
separated lean, braised, 3.5 oz	244	28	0	13.8	5.9	0
Ground						
extra lean, broiled, medium, 3.5 oz	256	25.4	0	16	6.4	0
lean, broiled, medium, 3.5 oz	272	24.7	0	18.5	7.3	0
regular, broiled, medium, 3.5 oz	289	24.1	0	20.7	8.1	0
Rib eye						
small end, separated lean and fat, broiled, 3.5 oz	295	25.4	0	20.6	8.7	0
small end, separated lean, broiled, 3.5 oz	225	28	0	11.6	4.9	0
large end, separated lean and fat, broiled, 3.5 oz	378	20.1	0	32.3	13.7	0
large end, separated lean, broiled, 3.5 oz	233	24.6	0	14.2	6.1	
Short ribs						
separated lean and fat, braised, 3.5 oz	471	21.6	0	42	17.8	0
separated lean, braised, 3.5 oz	295	30.8	0	18.1	7.7	0
Ribs, whole (ribs 6–12)						
separated lean and fat, broiled, 3.5 oz	362	21.5	0	30	12.7	0
separated lean, broiled, 3.5 oz	228	26	0	13	5.5	0

	Kcal	Pro	Cho	Fat	Sfa	Dfib
MEATS (*cont.*)						
Round bottom						
separated lean and fat, braised, 3.5 oz	261	29.8	0	14.8	5.7	0
separated lean, braised, 3.5 oz	222	31.6	0	9.7	3.4	0
Round, eye of						
separated lean and fat, roasted, 3.5 oz	243	26.8	0	14.2	5.8	0
separated lean, roasted, 3.5 oz	183	29	0	6.5	2.5	0
Round tip						
separated lean and fat, roasted, 3.5 oz	251	26.5	0	15.3	6.1	0
separated lean, roasted, 3.5 oz	190	28.7	0	7.5	2.8	0
Sausage, smoked, canned, 1 oz	89	4	0.7	7.6	3.2	0
Short loin T-bone steak						
separated lean and fat, broiled, 3.5 oz	324	24	0	24.6	10.2	0
separated lean, broiled, 3.5 oz	214	28.1	0	10.4	4.2	0
Short loin, tenderloin						
separated lean and fat, broiled, 3.5 oz	226	26	0	17.2	7	0
separated lean, broiled, 3.5 oz	204	28.3	0	9.3	3.6	0
Wedge-bone sirloin						
separated lean and fat, broiled, 3.5 oz	280	27.4	0	18	7.5	0
separated lean, broiled, 3.5 oz	208	30.4	0	8	3.6	0

	Kcal	Pro	Cho	Fat	Sfa	Dfib
MEATS (*cont.*)						
Lamb						
Leg						
separated lean and fat, roasted, 3.5 oz	237	15.6	0	20.9	11.7	0
separated lean, roasted, 3.5 oz	158	24.4	0	6	3.4	0
Loin chop						
separated lean and fat, broiled, 3.5 oz	255	15.6	0	20.9	11.7	0
separated lean, broiled, 3.5 oz	92	13.8	0	3.7	2.1	0
Rib chop						
separated lean and fat, broiled, 3.5 oz	273	13.5	0	23.9	13.4	0
separated lean, broiled, 3.5 oz	91	11.7	0	4.5	2.5	0
Shoulder						
separated lean, roasted, 3.5 oz	174	22.8	0	8.5	4.8	0
Pork						
Bacon						
Canadian, grilled, 2 slices	86	11.3	0.6	3.9	1.3	0
cured, broiled/pan fried, 3 medium pieces	109	5.8	0.1	9.4	3.3	0
Bacon pieces, bacon bits, Oscar Meyer, ¼ cup	21	2.6	0.2	1		

	Kcal	Pro	Cho	Fat	Sfa	Dfib
MEATS (*cont.*)						
Center loin						
separated lean and fat, braised, 3.5 oz	354	29.4	0	25.4	9.2	0
separated lean, braised, 3.5 oz	272	34.8	0	13.7	4.5	0
Ham, roasted, 3.5 oz	178	22.6	0	9	3.1	0
Ham patties, grilled, 1 patty	203	7.9	1	18.4	6.6	0
Leg						
separated lean and fat, roasted, 3.5 oz	294	25	0	20.7	7.5	0
separated lean, roasted, 3.5 oz	220	28.3	0	11	3.8	0
Loin						
separated lean and fat, braised, 3.5 oz	368	27.2	0	27.9	10.1	0
separated lean, braised, 3.5 oz	273	33	0	14.6	5	0
Loin blade						
separated lean and fat, roasted, 3.5 oz	364	21.1	0	30.5	10.9	0
separated lean, roasted, 3.5 oz	279	24.7	0	19.3	6.7	0
Rump						
separated lean and fat, roasted, 3.5 oz	274	26.6	0	17.8	6.5	0
separated lean, roasted, 3.5 oz	221	29.1	0	10.7	3.7	0
Shoulder						
separated lean and fat, roasted, 3.5 oz	326	22	0	25.7	9.3	0

	Kcal	Pro	Cho	Fat	Sfa	Dfib
MEATS (*cont.*)						
separated lean, roasted, 3.5 oz	244	25.4	0	15	5.2	0
Top loin						
separated lean and fat, braised, 3.5 oz	381	27.7	0	29.2	10.6	0
separated lean, braised, 3.5 oz	277	34.4	0	14.4	5	0
Veal						
Chuck, braised/pot roasted/stewed, 3 oz	200	23.7	0	10.9	5.2	0
Loin, braised/broiled, 3 oz	199	22.4	0	11.4	5.5	0
Variety Cuts						
Beef brains, 3.5 oz	160	11.1	0	12.5	2.9	0
Beef heart, 3.5 oz	175	28.8	0.4	5.6	1.7	0
Beef liver, 3.5 oz	161	24.4	3.4	4.9	1.9	0
Beef sweetbreads, 3.5 oz	272	22	0	19.7		0
Beef tongue, 3.5 oz	283	22.1	0.3	20.7	8.9	0
MEATS, LUNCHEON						
Beef						
chopped, smoked, 1 oz	38	5.7	0.5	1.3	0.5	0
loaved lunch meat, 1 slice	87	4.1	0.8	7.4	3.2	0

	Kcal	Pro	Cho	Fat	Sfa	Dfib
MEATS, LUNCHEON (*cont.*)						
Bologna						
beef, 1 slice	72	2.8	0.2	6.6	2.8	0
pork, 1 slice	57	3.5	0.2	4.6	1.6	0
turkey, 1 slice	60	3.9	0.6	4.5	1.4	0
Bratwurst, pork, 1 link	256	12	1.8	22	7.9	0
Braunschweiger, 1 slice	65	2.4	0.6	22	7.9	0
Chicken roll, light meat, 2 slices	90	11.1	1.4	4.2	1.2	0
Frankfurter						
beef, 1 frank	180	6.9	1	16.3	6.9	0
chicken, 1 frank	116	5.8	3.1	8.8	2.5	0
turkey, 1 frank	100	5.8	0.6	8.1	2.7	0
Ham						
cured, chopped, 1 slice	50	3.4	0.1	4	1.3	0
sliced, lean 5% fat, 1 slice	37	5.5	0.3	1.4	0.5	0
Honey loaf, 1 slice	36	4.5	1.5	1.3	0.4	0
Kielbasa, 1 slice	81	3.5	0.6	7.1	2.6	0
Knackwurst/knockwurst, 1 slice	209	8.1	1.2	18.9	6.9	0
Meat spread						
chicken, canned, 1 oz	55	4.4	1.5	3.3		
ham, 1 oz	100	5	4	6	1.8	
Pastrami, beef, 1 oz	99	4.9	0.9	8.3	3	0
Salami, 1 slice	76	2.9	0.4	6.9	3	0
Smoked link sausage, pork, 1 link	265	15.1	1.4	21.6	7.7	0
pork and beef, 1 link	229	9.1	1	20.6	9.2	0
Turkey breast meat, 1 slice	23	4.7	0	0.3	0.1	0
Turkey pastrami, 1 slice	80	10.4	0.9	3.5	1	0

	Kcal	Pro	Cho	Fat	Sfa	Dfib
MILK, YOGURT, MILK BEVERAGES, AND MILK BEVERAGE MIXES						
Milk						
Buttermilk, 8 fl oz	99	8.1	11.7	2.2	1.3	0
Low fat 1%, 8 fl oz	102	8	11.7	2.6	1.6	0
Low fat 2%, 8 fl oz	121	8.1	11.7	4.7	2.9	0
Skim, 8 fl oz	86	8.4	11.9	0.4	0.3	0
Whole 3.5%, 8 fl oz	150	8	11	8	4.9	0
Yogurt						
Low fat, 8 fl oz	144	11.9	16	3.5	2.3	0
Whole, 8 fl oz	139	7.9	10.6	7.4	4.8	0
Milk Beverages and Mixes						
Eggnog, nonalcoholic, 8 fl oz	342	9.7	34.4	19	11.3	0
Milk shake						
thick chocolate, 1 average	356	9.2	63.5	8.1	5	0
vanilla, 1 average	350	12.1	55.6	9.5	5.9	0
NUTS						
Almonds						
dry roasted, 1 oz	167	4.6	6.9	14.7	1.4	
oil roasted, 1 oz	176	5.8	4.5	16.4	1.6	
Cashews						
dry roasted, 1 oz	163	4.4	9.3	13.2	2.6	
oil roasted, 1 oz	163	4.6	8.1	13.7	2.7	
Coconut						
raw, 1 piece	159	1.5	6.9	15.1	13.4	
dried, flaked, sweetened, canned, 4 oz	505	3.8	46.6	36.1	32	

	Kcal	Pro	Cho	Fat	Sfa	Dfib
NUTS (*cont.*)						
Macadamia						
dry roasted, 1 oz	193	2.4	2.5	21.2	3.1	
oil roasted, 1 oz	204	2.1	3.7	21.7	3.3	
Mixed nuts						
dry roasted, 1 oz	169	4.9	7.2	14.6	2	
oil roasted, 1 oz	175	4.8	6.1	16	2.5	
without peanuts, oil roasted, 1 oz	175	4.4	6.3	16	2.6	
Peanut butter						
creamy/smooth, 1 tablespoon	95	4.6	2.5	8.2	1.4	
chunky style, 1 tablespoon	94	3.5	4.4	8	1.5	
Peanuts						
dry roasted, 1 oz	164	6.6	6	13.9	1.9	
oil roasted, 1 oz	165	7.6	5.3	14	1.9	
Pecans						
dry roasted, 1 oz	187	2.3	6.3	18.4	1.5	
oil roasted, 1 oz	195	2	4.6	20.2	1.6	
Pistachio						
dry roasted, 1 oz	172	4.2	7.8	15	1.0	
POULTRY						
Chicken						
Back, with skin, fried, ½ back	238	20	6.7	14.9	4	0
Breast						
with skin, fried, ½ breast	218	31.2	1.6	8.7	2.4	0
with skin, roasted, ½ breast	193	29.2	0	7.6	2.2	0

	Kcal	Pro	Cho	Fat	Sfa	Dfib
POULTRY (*cont.*)						
without skin, fried, ½ breast	161	28.8	0.4	4.1	1.1	0
without skin, roasted, ½ breast	142	26.7	0	3.1	0.9	0
Drumstick						
with skin, fried, 1 drumstick	120	13.2	0.8	6.7	1.8	0
with skin, roasted 1 drumstick	112	14.1	0	5.8	1.6	0
Leg						
with skin, fried, 1 leg	285	30.1	2.8	16.2	4.4	0
with skin, roasted, 1 leg	265	29.6	0	15.4	4.2	0
Thigh						
with skin, fried, 1 thigh	162	16.6	2	9.3	2.5	0
with skin, roasted, 1 thigh	153	15.5	0	9.6	2.7	0
without skin, roasted, 1 thigh	109	13.5	0	5.7	1.6	0
Wing						
with skin, fried, 1 wing	103	8.4	0.8	7.1	1.9	0
with skin, roasted, 1 wing	99	9.1	0	6.6	1.9	0
Unspecified type						
breast, oven roasted, Louis Rich, 1-oz slice	39	5.4	0.2	1.8	0.7	0
nuggets, breaded and frozen, Banquet, 3 oz	233	14	14	14		0

	Kcal	Pro	Cho	Fat	Sfa	Dfib
POULTRY (*cont.*)						
Turkey						
breast, barbecued, Louis Rich, 1 oz	39	6.2	0.5	1.3		0
Dark meat						
with skin, roasted, 3.5 oz	221	27.5	0	11.5	3.5	0
without skin, roasted, 3.5 oz	187	28.6	0	7.2	2.4	0
Light and dark meat						
with skin, roasted, 3.5 oz	208	28.1	0	9.7	2.8	0
without skin, roasted, 3.5 oz	170	29.3	0	5	1.6	0
Light meat						
with skin, roasted, 3.5 oz	197	28.6	0	8.3	2.3	0
without skin, roasted, 3.5 oz	157	29.9	0	3.2	1	0
Roll						
light and dark meat, 3.5 oz	149	18.1	2.1	7	2	0
SALAD DRESSINGS						
Low Calorie						
French, 1 tablespoon	22	0	3.5	0.9	0.1	0
Italian, 1 tablespoon	16	0	0.7	1.4	0.2	0
Russian, 1 tablespoon	23	0.1	4.5	0.7	0.1	0
Thousand island, 1 tablespoon	24	0.1	2.5	1.6	0.2	0

	Kcal	Pro	Cho	Fat	Sfa	Dfib
SALAD DRESSINGS (*cont.*)						
Regular						
Blue, 1 tablespoon	77	0.7	1.1	8	1.5	0
Buttermilk, 1 tablespoon	58	0.5	1.2	5.8	1	0
French, 1 tablespoon	67	0.1	2.7	6.4	1.5	0
Italian, 1 tablespoon	69	0.1	1.5	7.1	1	0
Mayonnaise, 1 tablespoon	57	0.1	3.5	4.9	0.7	0
Thousand island, 1 tablespoon	59	0.1	2.4	5.6	0.9	0
Vinegar and oil, homemade, 1 tablespoon	72	0	0.4	8	1.5	0
SAUCES AND CONDIMENTS						
Barbecue sauce, 1 tablespoon	12	0.3	2	0.3	0	0
Bernaise sauce, 1 tablespoon	263	3.1	6.6	25.6	15.7	0
Catsup, 1 tablespoon	16	0.3	3.8	0.1		0
Hollandaise sauce, 1 tablespoon	47	0.9	2.7	3.9	2.3	0
Horseradish, 1 tablespoon	6	0.2	1.4	0	0	0
Horseradish sauce, 1 tablespoon	54	0.1	2.3	4.9	0.8	0
Marinara sauce, 1 tablespoon	171	4.0	25.4	8.4	1.2	0
Mustard						
brown, 1 teaspoon	5	0.3	0.3	0.3	0	0
yellow, 1 teaspoon	4	0.2	0.3	0.2	0	0
Pizza sauce, Contadina, $\frac{1}{4}$ cup	40	0	5	2	0.2	0

	Kcal	Pro	Cho	Fat	Sfa	Dfib
SAUCES AND CONDIMENTS (*cont.*)						
Soy sauce, ¼ cup	30	3	4.9	0.1	0	0
Spaghetti sauce, 1 cup	272	4.5	39.7	11.9	1.7	0
with meat flavor, Prego, 1 cup	142	2.4	20.2	5.8		0
with mushrooms, 4 oz	133	1.8	19.8	5.2	0	0
Teriyaki sauce, bottled, 1 tablespoon	15	1.1	2.9	0	0	0
Tomato sauce, ½ cup	37	1.6	8.8	0.2	0	0
White cream sauce, 2 oz	59	0.7	3.8	4.5		0
SOUPS						
Canned, Condensed, Prepared with Water						
Asparagus, cream of, 1 cup	87	2.3	10.7	4.1	1	
Beef, Campbell's, 1 cup	71	4.9	9.6	1.5		
Beef noodle, 1 cup	84	4.8	9	3.1	1.2	
Broccoli, cream of, 1 cup	69	1.5	9.5	2.7		
Cheese, 1 cup	155	5.4	10.5	10.5	6.7	
Chicken and stars, Campbell's 1 cup	55	3.1	6.5	1.8		
Chicken broth, 1 cup	39	4.9	0.9	1.4	0.4	
Chicken and broth, Campbell's, 1 cup	44	1.4	7.4	1		
Chicken						
cream of, 1 cup	116	3.4	9.3	7.4	1.5	
gumbo, 1 cup	56	2.6	8.4	1.4	0.3	
noodle, 1 cup	75	4	9.4	2.5	0.7	
and rice, 1 cup	60	3.5	7.2	1.9	0.5	
vegetable, 1 cup	74	3.6	8.6	2.8	0.9	

	Kcal	Pro	Cho	Fat	Sfa	Dfib
SOUPS (*cont.*)						
Clam chowder						
Manhattan, 1 cup	78	4.2	12.2	2.3	0.4	
New England, 1 cup	95	4.8	12.4	2.9	0.4	
Consomme, with gelatin, 1 cup	29	5.4	1.8	0	0	
Garden vegetable, Campbell's, 1 cup	63	2.2	9.7	1.8		
Minestrone, 1 cup	83	4.3	11.2	2.5	0.5	
Mushroom, cream of, 1 cup	129	2.3	9.3	9	2.4	
Onion, 1 cup	57	3.8	8.2	1.7	0.3	
Pea, green, 1 cup	164	8.6	26.5	2.9	1.4	
Potato, cream of, 1 cup	73	1.7	11.5	2.4	1.2	
Tomato, 1 cup	86	2.1	16.6	1.9	0.4	
Tomato rice, 1 cup	120	2.1	21.9	2.7	0.5	
Turkey noodle, 1 cup	69	3.9	8.6	2	0.6	
Vegetable						
Campbell's, 1 cup	79	3.1	13.3	1.5		
vegetarian, 1 cup	72	2.1	12	1.9	0.3	
SPREADS (BUTTER, MARGARINE, MAYONNAISE)						
Butter, 1 teaspoon	36	0	0	4.1	2.5	0
Butter buds, 2 teaspoons, dry	12	0	2.9	0.1		
Margarine						
soft, 1 tablespoon	100	0	0	11	2	
stick, corn, 1 teaspoon	34	0	0	3.8	0.6	
tub, corn, 1 teaspoon	34	0	0	3.8	0.7	
Mayonnaise, 1 tablespoon	100	0.2	0.1	11.2	1.7	

	Kcal	Pro	Cho	Fat	Sfa	Dfib
SPREADS (BUTTER, MARGARINE, MAYONNAISE) (*cont.*)						
Miracle Whip, 1 tablespoon	69	0.1	1.7	6.9	1.1	
SUGARS, SYRUPS, AND OTHER SWEETENERS						
Honey, 1 tablespoon	64	0.1	17.3	0		
Jams/preserves, 1 tablespoon	54	0.1	14	0		
Jelly, 1 tablespoon	49	0	12.7	0		
Sugar						
brown, 1 cup	541	0	139.8	0	0	
white, 1 teaspoon	15	0	4	0	0	
white, 1 cup	770	0	199	0	0	
Sugar substitute						
Equal, 1 packet	4	0	1	0		
Sweet 'n Low, 1 packet	4	0	0.9	0		
Syrup						
cane and maple, 1 tablespoon	50	0	12.8	0		
corn, 1 tablespoon	59	0	15.4	0		
VEGETABLES, VEGETABLE PRODUCTS, AND VEGETABLE SALADS						
Asparagus						
boiled, ½ cup	22	2.3	4	0.3	0.1	
canned, ½ cup	24	2.6	3	0.8	0.2	
Avocado, 1 medium	306	3.6	12	30	4.5	4.7
Beans						
canned baked, B and M, ⅞ cup	330	16	49	8		
baked with honey, B and M, ⅞ cup	280	15	50	2		

	Kcal	Pro	Cho	Fat	Sfa	Dfib
VEGETABLES, VEGETABLE PRODUCTS, AND VEGETABLE SALADS (*cont.*)						
Beans, refried, 1 cup	270	15.8	46.8	2.7	1	
Beets, boiled, ½-cup slices	26	0.9	5.7	0	0	
Broccoli						
boiled, ½ cup	23	2.3	4.3	0.2	0	
with cheese sauce, Birds Eye, ½ cup	116	4.8	11.6	6.2	1.9	
Brussel sprouts						
boiled, ½ cup	30	2	6.5	0.3	0.1	1.4
Birds Eye, with cheese sauce, ½ cup	113	5	12.5	5.6	1.7	
Cabbage						
raw, ½ cup	8	0.4	1.9	0.1	0	0.4
boiled, ½ cup	16	0.8	3.5	0.2	0	
Carrots						
raw, 1 medium	31	0.7	7.3	0.1	0	1.1
boiled, ½ cup	17	0.5	4	0.1	0	0.9
Cauliflower						
raw, ½ cup	12	1	2.5	0.1	0	0
boiled, ½ cup	15	1.2	2.9	0.1	0	0.1
with cheese sauce, Birds Eye, ½ cup	114	4	11.7	6.1	1.9	
Celery, raw, 1 stalk	6	0.3	1.5	0.1	0	0.4
Chickpeas, canned, 1 cup	285	11.5	54.3	2.7	0.3	
Corn						
boiled, ½ cup	89	2.7	20.6	1.1	0.2	
canned, ½ cup	66	2.2	15.2	0.8	0.1	1.1
cream style, ½ cup	93	2.2	23.2	0.5	0.1	
Green beans						
boiled, ½ cup	22	1.2	4.9	0.2	0	1.1

	Kcal	Pro	Cho	Fat	Sfa	Dfib
VEGETABLES, VEGETABLE PRODUCTS, AND VEGETABLE SALADS (*cont.*)						
canned, ½ cup	13	0.8	3.1	0.1	0	0.0
Lentils						
1 cup	231	17.9	39.9	0.7	0.1	7.9
sprouts, 3.5 oz	101	8.8	821.3	0.5	0.1	
Mushrooms						
raw, ½ cup	9	0.7	1.6	0.2	0	
boiled, ½ cup	21	1.7	4	0.4	0	
Onions						
raw, ½ cup	27	0.9	5.9	0.2	0	0.6
boiled, ½ cup	29	1	6.6	0.2	0	
dehydrated flakes, ¼ cup	45	1.3	11.7	0.1	0	
Peas, boiled, ½ cup	67	4.3	12.5	0.2	0	3
Peppers, raw, ½ cup	12	0.4	2.7	0.2	0	0.6
Potatoes						
baked, with skin, 1 medium	220	4.7	51	0.2	0.1	
baked, without skin, 1 medium	145	3.1	33.6	0.2	0.1	
french fried, 10 pieces	158	2	20	8.3	2.5	
au gratin, from mix, ⅙ of 5.5-oz package	127	3.2	17.6	5.6	3.5	
Rice						
brown, 1 cup	232	4.9	49.7	1.2		
white, 1 cup	223	4.1	49.6	0.2		
Tofu, ½ cup	1183	19.9	5.4	11	1.6	
Spinach						
raw, ½ cup	6	0.8	1	0.1	0	0.9
boiled, ½ cup	21	2.7	3.4	0.2	0	1.7
Squash, all varieties, boiled, ½ cup	18	0.8	3.9	0.3	0.1	1

	Kcal	Pro	Cho	Fat	Sfa	Dfib
VEGETABLES, VEGETABLE PRODUCTS, AND VEGETABLE SALADS (*cont.*)						
Sweet potato						
baked, 1 medium	118	2	27.7	0.1	0	2.1
candied, 1 medium	144	0.9	29.3	3.4	1.4	
Tomato						
raw, 1 medium, canned, ½ cup	24	1.1	5.3	0.3	0	1.0
stewed, ½ cup	34	1.2	8.3	0.2	0	
whole, peeled, ½ cup	24	1.1	5.2	0.3	0	0.8
paste, ½ cup	110	5	24.7	1.2	0.2	

18

The New You

You have now read The Wellness Way to Weight Loss. Let's recap some of what you have learned.

WHY OTHER DIETS FAIL

Other diets fail because even though you may lose a tremendous amount of weight following their program, the weight comes right back on. This happens because the diets do not teach you to alter your eating habits. So as soon as you stop following their program or eating their special foods or drinking their liquid mixtures, you fall back on your old ways of eating and the pounds start piling back on.

This diet is different. As you follow the program you learn how to eat in the Wellness way. You learn what foods are good foods, what foods to avoid, and why. You learn you can eat foods everyone else eats and in normal amounts. You also learn that you, like everyone else, will slip off the diet but that occasional straying isn't disastrous for your weight loss.

The Wellness diet is also different in that you modify your

Fat Stat. As you follow the diet and exercise aerobically, your Fat Stat will be lowered. A lowered Fat Stat equals lower weight. It is your Fat Stat which ultimately determines how much you will weigh. Most of the other diets you have tried probably have not helped you modify your Fat Stat, another reason they have failed.

THE IMPORTANCE OF FIBER

Fiber is the cornerstone of the Wellness diet. A high fiber diet causes you to absorb less fat from the food you eat. The less fat you absorb the fewer calories you absorb. A high fiber diet will also help you decrease your risk of gastrointestinal problems such as colitis, hemorrhoids, and constipation. In addition, a high fiber diet helps to decrease your risk of cancer and heart disease.

EAT LESS FAT

The average American diet contains 37 percent fat. The recommended amount of fat in the diet is only 30 percent and only 10 percent of this amount should be saturated fat. The Wellness diet contains the proper amount of fat. Fat has the opposite effect from fiber; the less fat you eat the less your risk of heart disease and certain types of cancer. Also, the less fat you eat the easier it will be for you to lose weight. This is so because fat is a high-density food. In each gram of fat there are 9 calories, whereas each gram of protein or carbohydrate contains only 4 calories per gram. So fat contains many more calories per serving than any other food, and the less you eat of it, as soon as you obtain the minimal amount you need, the better.

EXERCISE

Exercise combined with the diet is the key to adjusting your Fat Stat. No one exercise is better than another. You can choose from a number of them, and as long as you exercise at least 20 to 30 minutes, 5 times a week, you will adjust your Fat Stat and you will lose weight.

THE DIET

The diet you should start on is the 1000-calorie diet. This will insure weight loss. As you lose the weight you desire you will gradually increase your calorie intake to the level that will allow you to maintain your weight at its ideal. By this time you will have learned about Wellness foods, how to read labels, how to dine out, and how to shop the Wellness way. Eating the Wellness way will become second nature. You will feel better, look better, and be well on your way to a Wellness life-style.

Bibliography

CHAPTER 2: WELLNESS: WHAT IS IT?

Pricilla D. Douglas, "Are Dieticians Ready for the Wellness Movement?" *Journal of the American Dietary Association* 1986: 92.
Jerry A. Johnson, "Wellness and Occupational Therapy," *American Journal of Occupational Therapy* 40 (1986): 753.
John V. Verner, "Ideas on Wellness," *North Carolina Medical Journal* 47 (1986): 355.

CHAPTER 3: THE FAT STAT

Dennis W. Remington, A. Garth Fisher, and Edward A. Parent, *How to Lower Your Fat Thermostat*. Provo, UT: Vitality House, 1988.

CHAPTER 4: THE UPS AND DOWNS OF WEIGHT LOSS WITHOUT WELLNESS

Geoffrey Cannon and Hetty Enizig, *Dieting Makes You Fat*. New York: Simon & Schuster, 1987.
Patricia Long, "Fat Chance," *Hippocrates* 5 (1989): 39.

Dennis W. Remington, A. Garth Fisher, and Edward A. Parent, *How to Lower Your Fat Thermostat*. Provo, UT: Vitality House, 1988.
Richard Trubo, "Fad Diets: Unqualified Hunger for Miracles," *Medical World News* 8 (1986): 44.

CHAPTER 5: WHY DO WE OVEREAT?

Stephen Langer and James F. Scheer, *Solve the Riddle of Weight Loss*. Rochester, VT: Healing Arts Press, 1989.

CHAPTER 6: FIBER: THE GREAT WARRIOR IN WEIGHT LOSS

Jane Brody, *Jane Brody's Nutrition Book*. New York: Bantam Books, 1981.

CHAPTER 7: FIBER AND DISEASE

Jane Brody, *Jane Brody's Nutrition Book*. New York: Bantam Books, 1981.
Marion J. Franz, "Your Fiber Guide," *Diabetes Forecast*, January 1988.
J. R. Varma, "Dietary Fiber: Individualizing the Prescription in Health and Sickness," *Consult* 28 (1988): 12.

CHAPTER 8: CARBOHYDRATES: THE GOOD, THE BAD, THE UNNECESSARY

Jane Brody, *Jane Brody's Nutrition Book*. New York: Bantam Books, 1981

CHAPTER 9: FATS: THE DELICIOUS BUT DANGEROUS FOODS

Jane Brody, *Jane Brody's Nutrition Book*. New York: Bantam Books, 1981.

CHAPTER 10: FATS AND DISEASE

Jane Brody, *Jane Brody's Nutrition Book*. New York: Bantam Books, 1981.
"Inform," *New Information on Health and Medicine*, September 1989.
Robert Stark, *Controlling Fat for Life*. Tuscon: Arizona Bariatric Physicians, 1986.
University of California Wellness Letter, 5 (1988): 1.

CHAPTER 11: PROTEIN: THE MEAT EATER'S MENTALITY

Jane Brody, *Jane Brody's Nutrition Book*. New York: Bantam Books, 1981.

CHAPTER 12: EXERCISE: ENERGIZING WEIGHT LOSS

Kenneth Cooper, *The Aerobics Program For Total Well-Being*. New York: Bantam Books, 1982.
Dennis W. Remington, A. Garth Fisher, and Edward A. Parent, *How to Lower Your Fat Thermostat*. Provo, UT: Vitality House, 1988.

CHAPTER 14: RECIPES FOR WELLNESS

Microwave Cooking Library™. Copies of the following books are available in bookstores and can be ordered, toll-free, by calling Cy DeCosse Incorporated at 1-800-328-3895 in the United States between 9 AM and 4 PM, Central Time.

Basic Microwaving
Recipe Conversion for Microwave
Microwaving Meats
Microwave Baking & Desserts
Microwaving Meals in 30 Minutes
Microwaving on a Diet
Microwaving Fruits & Vegetables
Microwaving Convenience Foods
Microwaving for Holidays & Parties
Microwaving for One & Two
The Microwave & Freezer
101 Microwaving Secrets
Microwaving Light & Healthy
Microwave Poultry & Seafood
Microwaving America's Favorites
Microwaving Fast & Easy Main Dishes
More Microwaving Secrets
Microwaving Light Meals & Snacks
Holiday Microwaving Ideas
Easy Microwaving Menus
Low Fat Microwaving
Cool, Quick Summer Microwaving
Ground Beef Microwave Meals

CHAPTER 15: THE WELLNESS BUYING GUIDE

Tips on Wise Food Selection. Dallas, TX: American Heart Association Grocery Guide, 1982.

CHAPTER 16: DINING OUT THE WELLNESS WAY

Dining Out: A Guide to Restaurant Dining. Dallas, TX: American Heart Association, 1984.

CHAPTER 17: FOOD VALUES

Jean A. T. Pennington, *Food Values of Portions Commonly Used,* 15th ed. New York: Harper & Row, 1989.

Index

GPSR Compliance

The European Union's (EU) General Product Safety Regulation (GPSR) is a set of rules that requires consumer products to be safe and our obligations to ensure this.

If you have any concerns about our products, you can contact us on ProductSafety@springernature.com

In case Publisher is established outside the EU, the EU authorized representative is:

Springer Nature Customer Service Center GmbH
Europaplatz 3
69115 Heidelberg, Germany

Batch number: 10822832

Printed by Printforce, the Netherlands